Building an Electronic Disease Register

Getting the computers

Alan Gillies

Nick Lowe

Radcliffe Medical Press

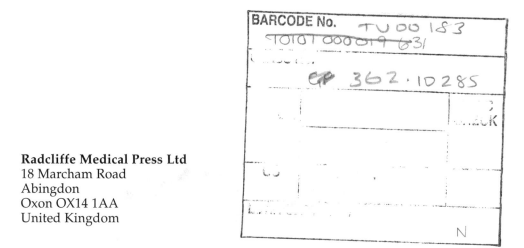
Radcliffe Medical Press Ltd
18 Marcham Road
Abingdon
Oxon OX14 1AA
United Kingdom

www.radcliffe-oxford.com
The Radcliffe Medical Press electronic catalogue and online ordering facility.
Direct sales to anywhere in the world.

© 2002 Alan Gillies, Bev Ellis and Nick Lowe

British Library Cataloguing in Publication Data

A catalogue record for this book is available from the British Library.

ISBN 1 85775 423 9

Typeset by Action Publishing Technology Ltd, Gloucester
Printed and bound by TJ International Ltd, Padstow, Cornwall

Contents

What this book is about   v
About the authors   vii
Acknowledgements   viii

Part One   The process of implementing an EDR   1

  1 What is an electronic disease register?   3
  2 Computerising patient records   7
  3 Managing the process of change   21

Part Two   Fylde PCG: a case study   51

  4 The case study and its context   53
  5 Establishing agreed policies across the PCG   61
  6 Implementing the policy   67
  7 Implementing the policy in an In Practice VISION practice   73
  8 Implementing the CHD policy in an EMIS practice   93

Part Three   Where do we go from here?   109

  9 Future PCG developments for coding CHD   111
10 Conclusions   125

Appendices   Further resources   129

Appendix A   VISION guidance for the NSF   131
Appendix B   The web site   147
Appendix C   HIP for CHD protocol in EMIS   149

Index   151

What this book is about

This book has two aims. The first is to demonstrate that computers can work for you and not the other way around. No, please don't laugh ... it really is possible. Computers can play a major role in improving patient health and patient care.

However, in order to achieve this, it is necessary to do a number of things:

- computerise patient records
- implement systems to process those records in accordance with best known practice and available evidence
- change working practices and procedures
- train staff to give them new skills
- manage the process of change.

Thus the second aim of the book is to show how to do these things in practice. We shall use the example of an electronic coronary heart disease register (CHD) to show how this may be achieved.

We shall draw upon a case study from a local primary care group (PCG) where we shall consider the implementation in two practices, with different proprietary general practice systems. We shall consider the example from the perspective of a GP and a practice manager.

How the book is organised

The first section of the book provides an overview of the process of implementing an electronic disease register and the issues involved.

The second part of the book shows how Fylde PCG have implemented their coronary heart disease register.

The third part of the book considers future developments, including the impact of the NSF CHD.

The Appendices include more information about products and services that may be helpful.

The clinical computer system suppliers inevitably modify and reconfigure their systems to meet the changing needs of the NHS. This means that practices may have slightly different versions or configurations from one another. This book uses specific examples from general practice in the UK (in 2001) and is intended to increase awareness of how the systems can be used to benefit PCG/Ts, practices and, not least, patients. Earlier versions of clinical software may not include all the features described – latest versions may offer enhanced features. Most of the features described are available on the majority of current systems from the main suppliers – if the descriptions do not exactly match your system, please refer to your current system manuals and training support teams.

About the authors

The book is the result of a collaboration between three authors each bringing their own perspective:

Professor Alan Gillies is Professor of Information Management at the University of Central Lancashire. He is an academic with 12 years experience of working with the NHS on information issues.

Beverley Ellis is Practice Manager with the Ash Tree House Surgery in Kirkham, Lancashire. The practice is an NHS Beacon site for informatics, and was one of the first users of the VISION system in the UK.

Dr Nick Lowe is a GP in Lytham, at the Holland House Surgery. He is an active member of the EMIS User Group and was responsible for the practice's award winning web site: www.lythamsurgery.co.uk.

The purpose of telling you this is not to blow our own trumpets, but rather to indicate the perspectives from which the authors come.

Acknowledgements

At the risk of sounding like an Oscar ceremony, this book has been made possible by the collaboration and co-operation of a wide range of people including, but not exclusively:

- Fylde PCG for giving permission to use them as a case study.
- The staff of Holland House Surgery and Ash Tree House Surgery.
- In Practice Systems and EMIS for their help in relation to the implementation sections.
- John Howard, Health Informatics Unit, UCLAN for the screen shots from the GPIMM and TNAMM tools.
- Magnus Hird at Blackpool PCG and Dr Hilary Devitt from Leeds NE PCG for contributing the CHD code matrix and content in Chapter 9. This is work still in progress (December 2000).

The authors wish to express their grateful thanks to all who have helped.

Part One

The process of implementing an EDR

Chapter 1

What is an electronic disease register?

The foundation for any patient records system are the records themselves. Traditionally, they have been held on paper, kept in brown envelopes and filed into a crude system by arranging them into alphabetical order within a filing cabinet:

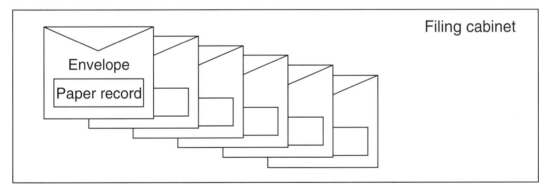

Schematic representation of a paper-based clinical records system.

A computerised record system may be viewed in a similar way:

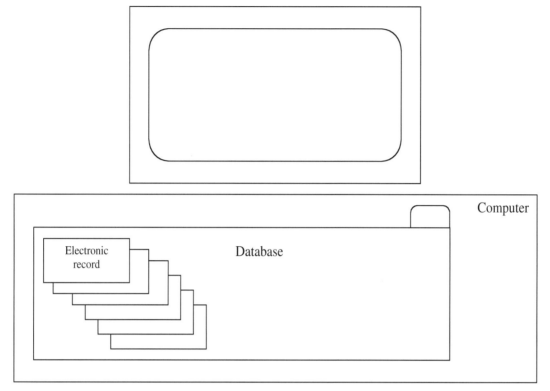

Schematic representation of an electronic patient records system.

However, the superficial similarity can be misleading. The paper-based system exists within a passive container. The database holding the electronic records is active, bringing with it the possibility of automating many information management functions.

At its simplest, the database management system allows us to sort the records in a wide range of ways:

- by surname
- by date of birth
- by home postcode etc.

The next function is the ability to filter records, i.e. to pull out a sample of the population with specific characteristics, e.g.

Women patients between the ages of 18 and 65

or

male patients in the age range 35–50 who are overweight, smoke and with a family history of CHD.

Whilst this can be done by manual inspection of paper records, for any significant population, the task is laborious and unreliable.

A traditional disease register is a collection of patients with specific characteristics. At its simplest, it might be regarded as a list of patients with a specific diagnosis. However, as healthcare moves towards prevention and health promotion, so disease registers are becoming prospective in identifying groups of patients considered 'at risk'.

Thus for CHD, factors identifying patients 'at risk' would include:

*   adverse Body Mass Index (BMI)
*   smoking
*   heavy drinking
*   diabetes
*   family history of CHD, and so on.

As disease registers become more and more prospective in nature, the need to make them electronic in order to keep them reliable and manageable becomes greater and greater.

A further dimension is provided by clinical governance. This places a clear requirement to demonstrate in a verifiable way that practice conforms to best evidence. The electronic system has the potential to both guide the clinician in accordance with protocols and guidelines and to audit practice.

Thus our electronic disease register may be regarded schematically as shown overleaf.

The clinical benefits obtainable from such a system promise to be a reliable, comprehensive, accurate and workable disease register capable of identifying and helping to manage 'at risk' patients, with consequent reductions in adverse events. The management benefits promise efficient use of resources, auditable performance monitoring, and improved health outcome measures.

However, as most of us know from bitter experience, computers rarely deliver nice, neat, simple solutions, and the reality is often complex, difficult and frustrating. In the rest of this book, we shall seek to minimise those frustrations and barriers and facilitate delivery of some of these promised benefits.

In the next chapter we shall consider the fundamentals of establishing a computerised patient records system, on which an electronic disease register depends.

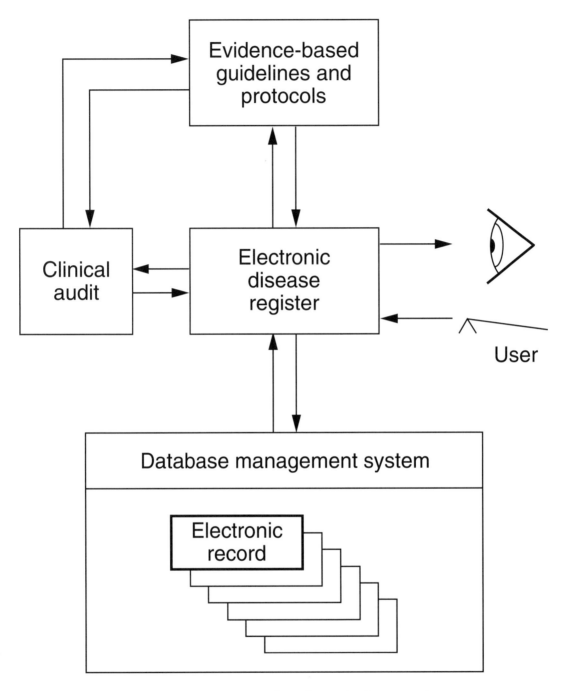

Schematic representation of an electronic disease register.

Chapter 2

Computerising patient records

The problem with computers

In spite of the upbeat tone of the previous chapter, the reality of computing within the NHS is rather different. People's experiences are often negative. This has been due to a number of factors, including the following.

Seven reasons for the current state of information in primary care

- The focus has been on the computers and not on the information.

- Computers have traditionally been time consuming to use, and worse they have not given back commensurate benefits.

- Staff have traditionally received little formal training.

- The NHS has been subject to frequent policy changes meaning that system designers have been shooting at a moving target.

- In primary care, much of the initial development was focused upon management developments to support fund holding rather than clinical developments.

- The English NHS woke up rather late to the need to share clinical data between practices. As early as 1993, some authors (alright, it was me, but not just me!) pointed out that the development of incompatible proprietary systems would inhibit progress.

- There has never been a policy of investing in clinician time to extend consultations to allow them to enter data during already short consultations.

There have also been a number of myths that have contributed to the current, less than ideal, state.

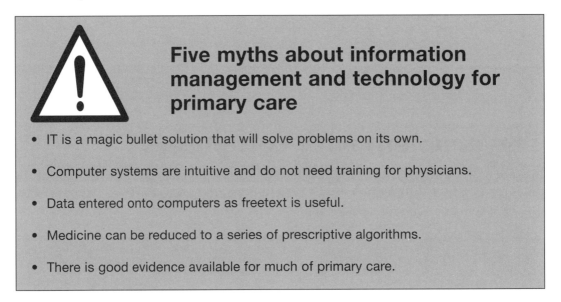

Five myths about information management and technology for primary care

- IT is a magic bullet solution that will solve problems on its own.

- Computer systems are intuitive and do not need training for physicians.

- Data entered onto computers as freetext is useful.

- Medicine can be reduced to a series of prescriptive algorithms.

- There is good evidence available for much of primary care.

This has led to a common perception that computers are more trouble than they are worth, a view that the author has characterised as the elephant view of health information systems.

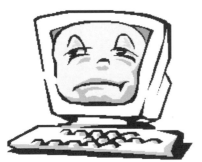 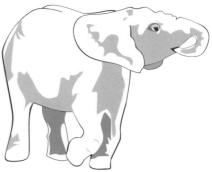

Spot the similarity?

We feed them both, most of what we feed in disappears, and the rest when it comes out is generally a pile of dung!

It may surprise the reader to learn that, in most cases, one of the authors (AG) believes that computers really are more trouble than they are worth. However, before you stop reading, the answer lies in better usage of the computers, not abandoning them altogether.

Making computers work for you

Many people have expressed the view that they are working for their computers, rather than the other way around. In 1992, AG was faced with the challenge of demonstrating to the Home Office that it was worth spending money on computerising the document production functions of a probation service.

In order to analyse this problem, we looked at the way in which computers could be used. We produced a model of computer usage for this context.

The model identified six distinct stages of development of the usage of the technology:

Phase 0 – Learning Initially, there is a 'learning' process associated with implementation of the document production facilities. Net benefits will actually be negative as office productivity drops. This involves not only getting used to the new physical environment and facilities but also involves disruption to tasks and dislocation in the organisational relationships with document production and delivery falling behind the previous schedules.

Phase 1 – Direct replacement Once learning has taken place, productivity recovers but the overhead, associated with new facilities implies that net benefits are likely to remain negative. For example, document checking and distribution remain as they were prior to the introduction of new facilities.

Phase 2 – Limited use of new technology The new features of document production available are explored by the operatives but, at this stage, use of such features is likely to be limited to the simpler aspects. At this stage net benefits are still likely to be zero. Tasks are still likely to take longer as document-checking procedures continue to rely on past experience. Very little organisational benefit is likely to occur as distribution of documents continues to conform to previous patterns.

Phase 3 – Extended use of new technology In this next phase, operatives begin to make use of advanced features such as style sheets, standard documents, spell checkers, etc. Operatives are able to manipulate the technology more speedily and effectively. Tasks are completed in a more professional manner. However, the time to set up standard documents and style sheets is likely to imply that document production is still delayed, causing some organisational dislocation.

Phase 4 – Automation of document production In this phase, operatives become familiar with macros and other advanced features. Increasingly, however, more effort has to be put into training for offices that find the complexity more demanding each time for the additional benefit obtained. Thus we see that the net benefit curve, steep in the middle phases, begins to level off. However, each individual task will take less time to perform and the degree of organisational benefit will improve.

Phase 5 – Integration The final stage involves the integration of document production. Retrieval of information from databases into documents, diagrams and charts, and e-mail facilities can all be integrated to hasten and automate the document production process to the full. Facilities such as e-mail and fax allow organisational integration to take place and improve the operation of the organisation.

In that study, it was suggested that net benefits do not accrue until Phase 3. In the next chapter we shall apply this kind of analysis to primary care information management.

The reality of most people's experience is that they never get past the stage where the net benefits are negative. They become discouraged and disillusioned, and give up. This is partly due to false expectations raised by management and systems suppliers.

A more realistic message of benefits accruing only after initial hard work and investment is often surprisingly well received by practitioners, welcoming its integrity and realism. However, real progress only comes when this reality is recognised by management and suitable resources are invested to get practices and PCGs to the stage of delivering real benefits in economic and health terms.

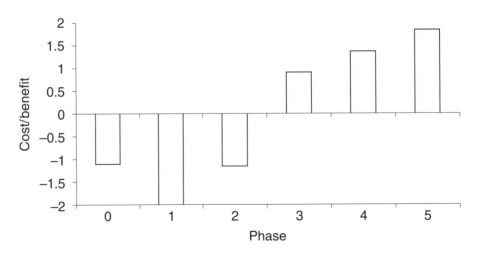

Cost benefit of IT.

The crucial issue of coding

Clinical codes are dull, boring and incomprehensible. People who talk about clinical codes at dinner parties are equally dull, boring and incomprehensible. (Yes I have been to dinners like that … it's where male doctors assert their masculinity by arguing that mine's bigger than yours, and they're talking about hard disks. Honestly!)

Unfortunately, clinical codes in general and Read Codes in particular are also essential for computerised patient records. To consider why this is so, compare the way that people talk and the way that computers talk.

People use natural language to communicate and to describe things. It has the advantage of being known to everyone, very flexible, able to express shades of opinion and fuzziness. It may also be accompanied by lots of hand waving! However, from the computer's point of view it is complex, inconsistent and requires a great deal of contextual information to interpret ambiguities.

Computers ultimately communicate using binary. These days we can turn binary into all sorts of things but ultimately they must be transferable into discrete bits.

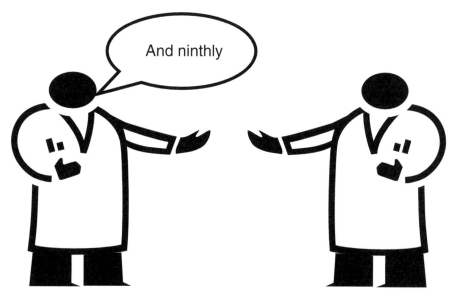

The way people talk.

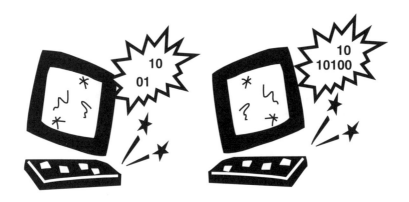

How computers talk.

One of the most common examples of this domestically is the use of digital audio technology on CDs. To do this, an audio signal must be 'digitised':

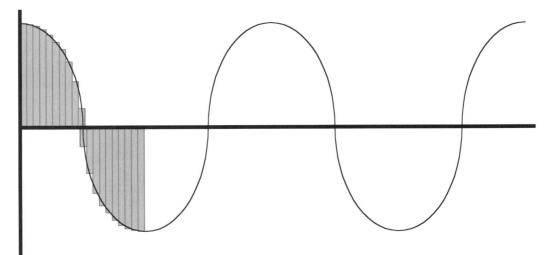

In the same way, many clinical matters, particularly diagnosis, are not discrete but have a degree of uncertainty attached to them. If you want to give a computer a headache, then tell it you've got a bit of a headache! There are many complexities that are difficult for the computer to deal with. Some of these include:

- variations in judgements between clinicians
- patients' interpretation of symptoms which may be quite wrong
- patients not revealing symptoms because of embarrassment
- complex interactions between multiple problems.

Clinical coding will not address all of these issues, but it does at least provide a way of representing a human diagnosis in a form that the computer can swallow.

Clinical coding systems

A variety of coding systems have been developed to meet different needs. Some of the principal systems have included:

Coding system	Developed for	Target audience
ICD9, ICD10	CDC/WHO	Epidemiology
Read	NHS	UK primary care
SNOMED	College of American Pathologists	Pathology

Each coding system may be thought of as a different medical language (sometimes they are known as medical vocabularies). As might be expected each has developed in accordance with the needs of its target audience. The same is true of languages. For example, Finnish, famed for being the most inaccessible of all European languages has no word for sandwich box because there is no such concept.

Also like languages, the systems have some quaint idiosyncrasies. One of my favourite idiosyncrasies within Read Codes arises from its incorporation at an early stage of codes based upon an American medico-legal system. Although sadly now marked as officially obsolete, codes for such everyday occurrences in the NHS as 'accidental poisoning occurring in an opera house' and 'judicial execution in an electric chair' may still be found by the diligent searcher.

In *Information and IT for Primary Care* (1999), AG suggests five reasons why coding is essential:

- codes provide unambiguous information suitable for computer processing
- codes allow standard morbidity data to be collected across a PCG population
- codes allow the definition and implementation of standard clinical guidelines and protocols across the practices of a PCG
- codes allow the collection of standard datasets for performance monitoring and clinical governance
- coding facilitates comparison between and within PCGs.

However, achieving the desired outcomes in the latter four cases is not straight forward. Coding has been invented because of the shortcomings in computers: but it is the human part of the process that has to adapt and this can be tricky.

Put simply, for coding to work:

> **Coding must be universal and consistent across the target population and the target condition.**

In the past, even when the target population has been a single practice, this has proved problematic. In the future, for the targets set in the New NHS White Paper, and in the goals set out above, the population may be the whole of the country (usually England, Scotland, Wales or Northern Ireland – the NHS rarely operates consistently in different parts of the UK) and regularly will be the whole of a PCG or PCT with up to 250 000 patients. This is a tall order, to say the least.

In this book, we shall focus upon Read Codes, although it is worth noting that the NHS is currently taking part in a project to combine the Read and SNOMED classification systems.

Read Codes

Read Codes were developed by Dr James Read, hence the name. They are a set of coded terms for use in clinical practice. They have a number of key features which make them the standard system for clinical coding in the UK primary care NHS:

- Read Codes were developed for primary care
- the codes are arranged in a hierarchical structure, so that an extensive clinical terminology can be readily accessed and used by computer software
- Read Codes are updated every 3 months, except for drugs which are updated every month
- Read Codes can be cross referenced to all other major systems, e.g. ICD, OPCS, BNF, ATC, etc.
- coding only works if everyone talks the same language, Read Codes are the UK NHS standard, therefore all other reasons are redundant.

There are in fact a number of versions of Read Codes. They were initially developed in the mid-1980s, as the 4-Byte Set for use in general practice. This first version provided a terminology for describing relevant clinical summary and administrative data. It is known as the 4-Byte Set since each code is four characters long.

The codes were subsequently adapted for use in hospitals, and were extended to allow more detail, leading to Version 2 of the Read Codes that was released in 1990. To accommodate extra detail, an additional alphanumeric character was added to the Read Code (5-Byte Sets – Version 1 and Version 2).

The history of these versions is summarised opposite in a table adapted from the NHSIA's guide to coding.

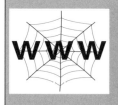

WWW link

At www.radcliffe-oxford.com/edr you will find links to the NHS Information Authority web site, which provides much more information about Read Codes.

4-Byte Set	The original version of the Read Codes was developed for GPs in the mid-1980s. In this version, Read Codes consist of only four alphanumeric characters. The files are much smaller than those in later versions, and contain fewer codes. This version contains approximately 40 000 codes. Text descriptions consist of up to 30 characters. 'Keys', which may be entered by users to select a group of related clinical terms, are four characters long.
5-Byte Version 1	This version was developed to include specific functions for cross-references to central returns for hospitals, as well as providing functionality for GPs. Read Codes are extended to five alphanumeric characters, allowing a 5-level hierarchy. Text descriptions still consist of up to 30 characters and keys are four characters long.
	The files were originally cross-referenced to the classifications of the Office of Population Censuses and Surveys for procedures [4th Revision (OPCS-4)] and the International Statistical Classification of Diseases and Related Health Problems for diagnoses (ICD-9, and from 1995, ICD-10). Maps are now maintained to OPCS-4 and ICD-10 only.
5–Byte Version 2	The codes are identical to 5-Byte Version 1, but text descriptions are extended to include 60- and 198-character versions, and keys are extended to 10 characters. A new code (the term code) allows more than one textual description of a Read-coded concept to be labelled and a 'preferred term' to be indicated.
	The Version 2 Read Codes also support cross-mapping to mandated classifications, including ICD-9 (up to 1995), ICD-10 (from 1995 onwards) and OPCS-4. Mappings to ICD-10 and OPCS-4 are currently maintained.

History of Read Code versions.

Clinical Terms Version 3 (CTV3) was developed as a result of the Clinical Terms Projects, which ran from 1992 to 1995 and was first released in 1994. This version introduced a new, more complex structure, allowing greater coverage and flexibility.

CTV3 is the current version of Read, and has been heavily pushed by the NHS IMG and NHSIA. They cite the following benefits for this version:

- it permits future changes in terminology to be evolutionary, by using a structure which can cope with new perspectives, details and functions demanded of the codes
- it allows multiple perspectives of the same concepts (to be equally useful for nursing, general practitioners (GPs), central returns, specialists etc.), and
- it produces more accurate and complete cross-mappings to other classifications.

In practice, in spite of these benefits, the most commonly used version of Read remains the 5-Byte Version 2 codes. With many clinicians still coming to terms with the basic principles of coding, another change appears to be a step too far.

With a further change to a combined SNOMED/Read system in the medium term, Version 3 may never be fully implemented.

To see how Read works in practice, let's consider a concrete example.

Consider, for example, ischaemic heart disease (IHD). We shall use Version 2 to illustrate it because it is still the most commonly used form of Read Codes.

In Read Code speak, a simple letter 'G' represents the circulatory system. Add a '3' to make a 'G3' code and we get to a code for IHD. Add more numbers and we get more detail. If we carry on adding more numbers to our example it goes as follows:

Circulatory system	G
IHD	G3
Acute myocardial infarction	G30
Anterior acute myocardial infarction	G301
Acute anteroseptal myocardial infarction	G3011

To see why we might even attempt this, let's look at another example.

How computers can help us manage IHD

The latest National Service Framework (NSF) on CHD advocates that:

'Every primary care team should ensure that all those with heart failure are receiving a full package of appropriate investigation and treatment, demonstrated by clinical audit data no more than 12 months old.'[1]

The computer can help us to:

- identify patients who fall into an at risk category
- generate letters to call those patients in for consultations
- monitor attendance at such consultations
- guide the clinician in the use of appropriate protocols
- record results from tests at the time of consultation
- record results from tests analysed after the consultation
- monitor incidence of adverse events amongst the target population
- record morbidity amongst the target population
- provide evidence for clinical governance
- provide evidence of the effectiveness of such treatments.

Key stages of this process will only happen if accurate and consistent electronic health records are held.

For example, if we consider the criteria for placing a patient in the at risk group, then we may identify a series of risk factors, e.g:

- overweight or obese
- smoking
- family history of heart disease
- previous adverse event etc.

The principle of a coding system is that it is hierarchical. The code for IHD is therefore G3 and all codes starting with G3 followed by more characters is simply a more detailed description of IHD.

However, the nature of medicine is such that sometimes it is not possible to define everything in a nice hierarchical tree. For example, in the case of IHD, there are a number of 'associated codes' that need to be added to cover all risk factors, e.g:

- CHD monitoring (662N)
- angina control (662K)

[1] Department of Health (2000) *National Service Framework for Coronary Heart Disease: modern standards and service models.* DoH, London.

- ECG shows myocardial infarction (322)
- ECG shows myocardial ischaemia (322)

Work done in local practices in Lancashire has been published.[2]

Age breakdown of patients with a Code for IHD (G3 or associated Codes*)

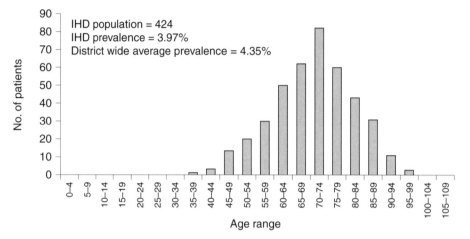

IHD population = 424
IHD prevalence = 3.97%
District wide average prevalence = 4.35%

* Associated codes = 662N CHD Monitoring; 662K Angina Control; 322% ECG shows MI; 323% Myocardial Ischaemia; 6625 Cardiac Drug Side-Effects; 6626 Cardiac Treatment Changed; 662D Cardiac DIS Treatment Started; 662E Cardiac DIS Treatment Stopped; 662J Cardiac Drug Monitoring; 662Z Cardiac Disease Monitoring NOS; 14A3 H/O Myocardial Infarction; 14A4 H/O Infarction >60.

Patients with a recording of IHD and a BP recording (246%) in the last 12 months*

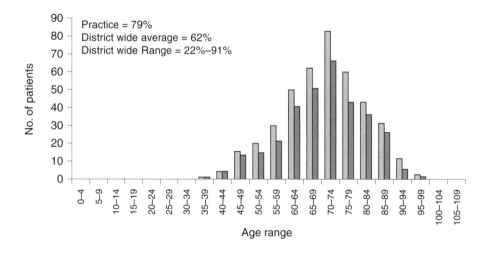

Practice = 79%
District wide average = 62%
District wide Range = 22%–91%

[2] Kumari N and Neild P (2001) Linking IHD. Data Quality and Clinical Audit in Primary Care: 'Improving patients' care … not judging patients' care'. *ePHI*. **1**: 1.

The figures opposite are examples of the results that have been generated. The Read Codes that the queries are extracting are listed below the graph. On each graph the district wide range is shown. The aim of this is to encourage practices to attempt to achieve those results at the higher end of the range, and the authors of this study advocate that if one practice can achieve a high result, it is possible for all practices to attempt to also achieve this, through good practice.

The first problem is that it may not always be obvious that a risk factor should be included. Increasingly, this is being addressed by the production of standard templates including specified codes for the National Service Frameworks (NSF) and other key areas. However, clinicians who may well regard this as an intrusion into their clinical autonomy may resist the imposition of such standards.

The advent of clinical governance may further increase resistance if people think that this sort of information might be taken down and used in evidence against them.

Having looked at some of the things we want to achieve, in the next chapter we will consider how we can get there, using three complementary approaches to managing the change which practices need to undergo.

Chapter 3

Managing the process of change

GPIMM: a strategic model for improving information management

Moving to electronic health records is not a simple or trivial process, as anyone who has been involved will agree. The real issues are not about the computers or codes at all, but about the changes in practice and process which are required.

There often appears to be a kind of information nirvana, as elusive as the pot of gold at the end of the rainbow.

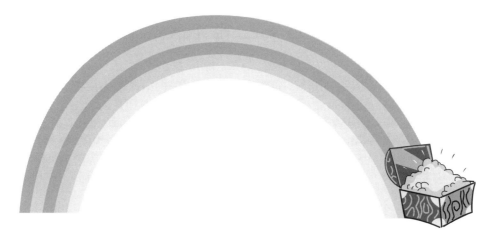

Electronic health records: unattainable nirvana?

However, it is possible to identify a series of key stages on the way to reaching this information nirvana, which may seem more attainable.

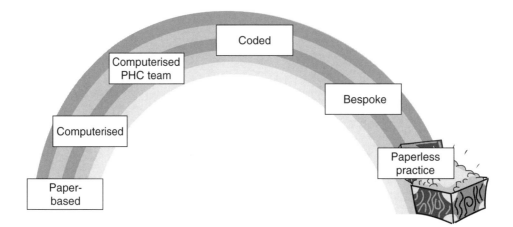

Five attainable steps from paper-based to paperless practice.

This approach is based around a model known as GPIMM, which stands for General Practice Information Maturity Model.

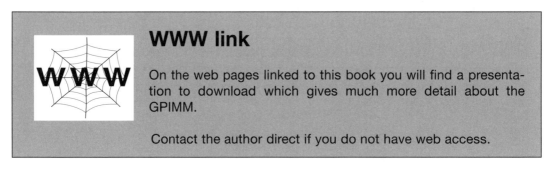

WWW link

On the web pages linked to this book you will find a presentation to download which gives much more detail about the GPIMM.

Contact the author direct if you do not have web access.

The idea of maturity model is based upon the capability maturity model (CMM) developed by the Software Engineering Institute (SEI) of Carnegie Mellon University. The SEI CMM was developed for the US Department of Defense to model the maturity of quality processes within their software suppliers.

The SEI maturity model is defined as a five-level framework for how an organisation matures its software processes from ad hoc, chaotic processes to mature, disciplined software processes.

SEI (1995) describes the levels indicated in the table at the top of the next page.

Level	Designation	Description
1	Initial	The organisation has undefined processes and controls
2	Repeatable	The organisation has standardised methods facilitating repeatable processes
3	Defined	The organisation monitors and improves its processes
4	Managed	The organisation possesses advanced controls, metrics and feedback
5	Optimising	The organisation uses metrics for optimisation purposes

Five levels of the SEI CMM (after SEI, 1995).

The SEI CMM is questionnaire-based. Questions are divided into 'essentials' and 'highly desirable'. To achieve a given level, an organisation must attain 90% 'yes' answers to essential questions and 80% 'yes' answers to highly desirable questions. The model is shown schematically below.

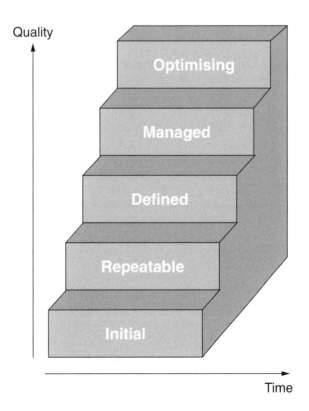

Schematic view of the SEI Capability Maturity Model.

The key characteristics of the SEI CMM that are utilised in the GPIMM model are:

- removal of a binary classification into 'quality' or 'not quality'
- definition of characteristics to define key stages of maturity
- definition of key actions to define how to move from each level to the next
- use of a questionnaire to facilitate analysis of current maturity.

A similar approach was used in the study described in the previous chapter to illustrate how benefits do not accrue until a certain level of development is reached. The GPIMM model describes information management maturity levels for primary care. Put more simply, it is a model of how well developed your information processes are.

It is based around five primary maturity levels, with an additional zeroth level for non-computerised practices.

The maturity levels are summarised in the table below.

Many practices are still at Levels 1 and 2, even after up to ten years of computing experience. This provides a significant barrier to clinical practice developments. The reality is that unless practices have procedures at Level 4 or above, they will not be able to realise significant clinical benefits from their systems, and the effort that they have to put in will not be matched by the benefits.

Level	Designation	Description
0	Paper-based	The practice has no computer system
1	Computerised	The practice has a computer system. It is used only by the practice staff
2	Computerised PHC team	The practice has a computer system. It is used by the practice staff and the PHC team, including the doctors
3	Coded	The system makes limited use of Read Codes
4	Bespoke	The system is tailored to the needs of the practice through agreed coding policies and the use of clinical protocols
5	Paperless	The practice is completely paperless, except where paper records are a legal requirement

Levels of the GPIMM.

The GPIMM framework provides a means for helping practices develop further to improve the usage of their systems. It should be noted that development will not, in many cases, require investment in new systems, but extract greater benefit from existing systems.

At Level 0, the practice is entirely based upon paper records. According to official statistics, by 1998 this was less than 2% of practices.

At Level 1, the computer has arrived. Typically, it is used in a limited way by administrative staff to assist in income generation by monitoring items for which the practice receives re-imbursement. Crucially, it is not used by clinicians in the consultation.

At Level 2, the computer is used by clinicians in a limited way. The practice has started to use the computer to store clinical information. However, the information is stored in freetext, making it simply an electronic notepad system. None of the advantages cited earlier can be realised whilst information is stored in this way.

At Level 3, the practice has started to code clinical information. Coding will be limited. The practice may not yet have fully formed policies to ensure that coding is consistent. Some benefits may be realised, but a lot of work remains to be done.

At Level 4, coding is well established as are policies to ensure codes are consistent and compatible with PCG/T standards to allow the practice to take part in local initiatives with other practices. At this stage, the system starts to deliver benefits greater than the effort required to make it work.

At Level 5, the practice is effectively operating in electronic fashion. Future developments are in the areas of continuous improvement and links with other agencies.

The GPIMM framework allows you to audit your practices and to define information strategies for each one, providing a structure improvement process to get practices to the required level.

The maturity level may be assessed through an audit, based around a computerised questionnaire. The questionnaire considers five areas to assess maturity:

- *computerisation* – this is simply a filter to identify those practices that remain paper-based
- *personnel usage* – this section looks at the impact of the system upon the practice. Systems used only by practice staff are severely limited in their usefulness.
- *coding* – this section is crucial. It considers not just the extent of coding, but the quality of coding through the extent of policies and consultation underpinning coding practice.
- *system usage* – this section is concerned with the impact that the system has upon the working methods of the practice. It measures the extent to which the system works for the practice and not the other way around
- *Electronic Patient Records* – this section is concerned with the implementation of the Electronic Patient Record. It considers how far the Electronic Patient Record is realised both inside and outside the practice.

GPIMM is a model designed for PCGs and PCTs. However, it evolved from a simpler single practice audit tool. We shall illustrate its use for a single practice using a simplified version of the model.

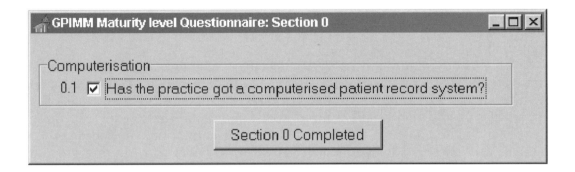

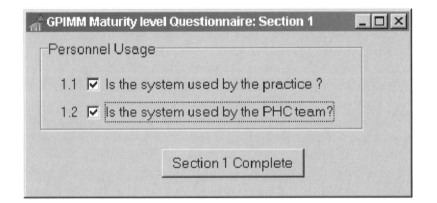

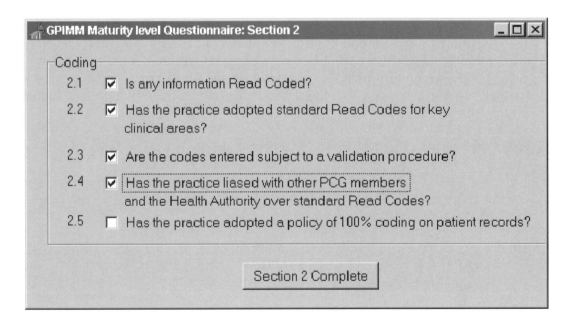

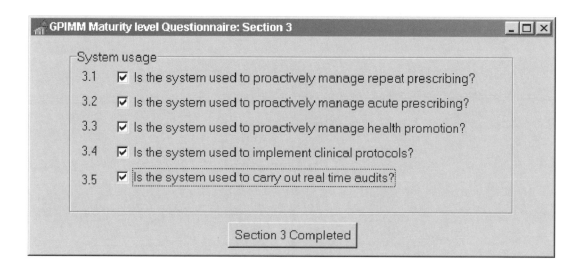

Early work with the GPIMM quickly highlighted the need for improvements in the information maturity of practices.

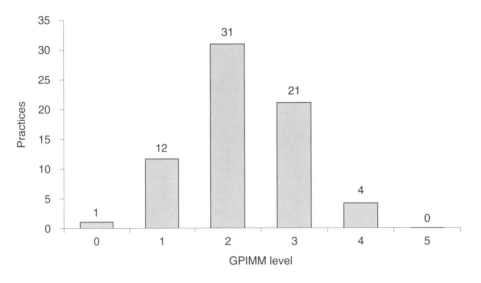

Typical PCG practice profile in terms of GPIMM ca. 1998.

The GPIMM allows us to define not only the current status of practices, but also a structured practice development path which will provide information strategies to bring each practice up to the required information maturity level to play a full role in the PCG information system.

We shall use a typical if somewhat traditional practice as a case study to help us.

Case Study Practice

This is a practice of 12,000 patients with five doctors, based in a suburban New Town area. The practice is based in a purpose built health centre behind a large super-market. The practice prides itself on the quality of care provided to its patients. It could be summarised as a 'traditional' practice with a stable staff. Their patient list is closed. They have never been a fund holding practice.

They are currently using an In-Practice Systems computer system. The system is based around the text-based VAMP Medical System with additional modules for items of service. The practice is linked to the health authority for items of service information.

The current usage of the system is limited. The doctors do not use the system during consultations. Instead, paper notes are used. Information from the paper notes is then entered on to the system at a later date by practice staff. Acute prescriptions are issued manually during consultations.

> Similarly, information is extracted from incoming letters by two medical secretaries, who enter key information on to the computer system. None of the information is currently coded.
>
> The practice manager is unhappy with the current situation and would like to move to a system making much greater use of the computer.

The responses to the maturity model questionnaire for this practice are given below.

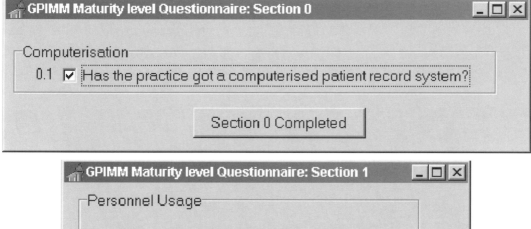

The system automatically logs the practice at Level 1 because of the non-involvement of the doctors. However, we can use the further facilities of the GPIMM-CAPA to make recommendations for practice improvement.

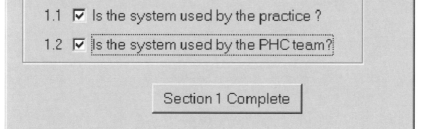

The report produced by entering 'Produce Report' gives the key tasks to be carried out in order to improve information maturity.

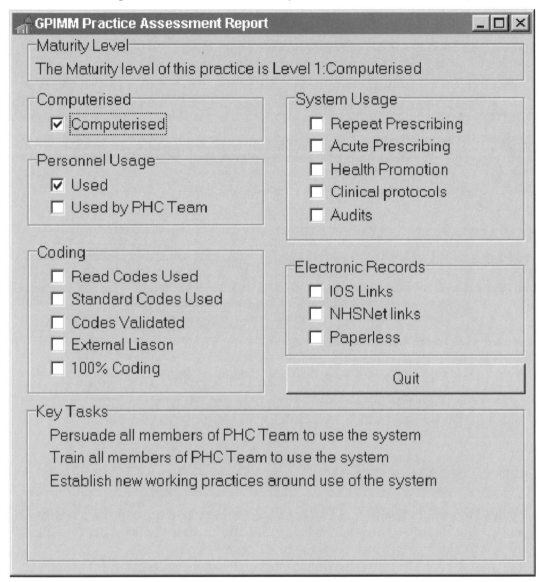

Each level of the GPIMM requires a major change in working practices. It is generally recommended that it should not be attempted to develop practices at a rate of more than one level per year.

Therefore, with practices such as this it is necessary to implement a long-term action plan to bring their information to the level required by the PCG. Each year, a GPIMM audit will be needed to check progress against the plan.

The plan for this practice, audited in 1999, is shown in the table below.

Year	GPIMM level	Tasks to be carried out
1999	1	• Persuade doctors and other PHC workers to use system in consultations • Train PHC team in use of system • Establish new working practices based around use of the system
2000	2	• Persuade all staff to use Read Codes • Train all staff in use of Read Codes • Discuss scope and nature of coding within practice • Liaise with PCG over coding standards • Implement codes within agreed scope
2001	2*	• Implement PCG coding standards with training • Implement practice defined protocols for diagnosis and prescribing with training • Implement computer based health promotion policy with training • Implement real-time audits with training
2002	4	• Move all records to electronic form • Agree coding standards with external bodies • Ensure system meets requirements for connection to NHSNet • Make paper records for legal requirements
2003	5	• Carry out audit to ensure that Level 5 is reached • Implement a culture of continuous monitoring and improvement

*To meet the requirements of Level 3, the practice would have to have implemented computerised repeat prescribing by this year. Once this is achieved, Level 3 will be attained early in 2001.

GPIMM is now encapsulated within a PCG(T) management information system, which keeps track of all the practices within a PCG, PCT or group of PCTs. This system is illustrated below.

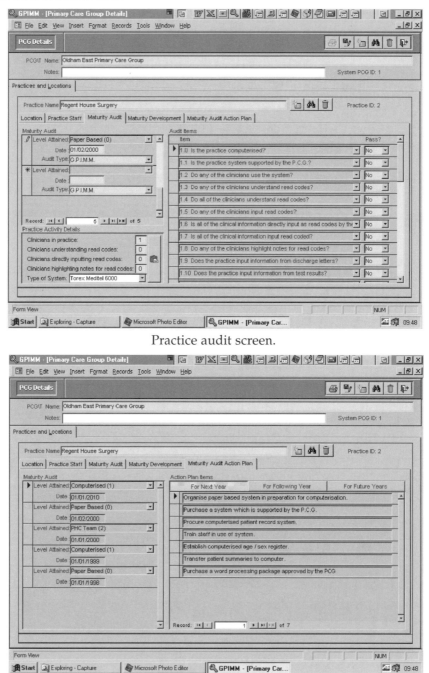

Practice audit screen.

Practice action screen.

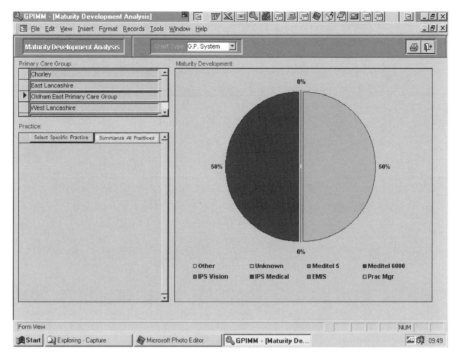

PCG practice systems profile report.

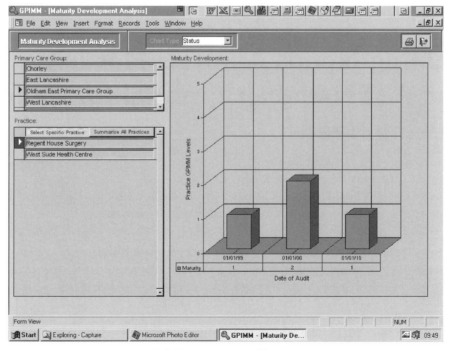

PCG practice profile.

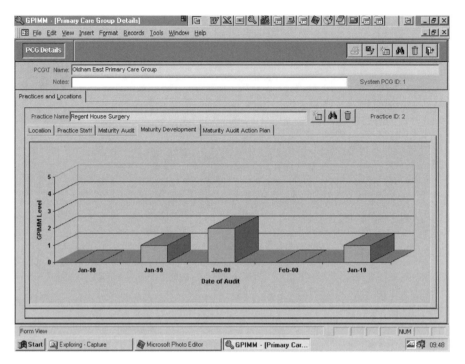

Individual practice profile over time.

Training Needs Analysis Maturity Model (TNAMM): a model for defining training needs

It has already been noted that one of the barriers to more effective use of IT to provide better information is the lack of training.

In order to deliver the process improvement defined by GPIMM it is also necessary to ensure that the personnel involved have the required skills.

For each level of GPIMM, required levels of competency have been defined for the key players in primary care, GPs, nurses, managers and administrators. Competencies are defined at one of five levels building on work by Dreyfus.[3]

---

[3] Dreyfus H and Dreyfus SE (1980) *A five-stage model of the mental activities involved in directed skill acquisition.* Unpublished report supported by the US Air Force Office of Scientific Research (Contract F49620-79-C-0063), University of California at Berkeley.

In this way, a training needs matrix may be defined for each GPIMM level:

Role	GP	Nurse	Manager	Administrator
Competency 1	Required level	Required level	Required level	Required level
Competency 2	Required level	Required level	Required level	Required level
Competency 3	Required level	Required level	Required level	Required level
Competency 4	Required level	Required level	Required level	Required level
Competency 5	Required level	Required level	Required level	Required level

The skills of the staff may then be audited against that required for the current or target GPIMM level.

Training may then be tailored to ensure that the capability of each person is that required to meet the needs of the organisation.

Consider the schematic profile below.

The member of staff concerned has more than the required skills in competencies 5, 7, 8, 15 and 16. They have the required skills in competencies 1–4, 14, 17–20. However, they do require training in competencies 6, 9, 10, 11, 12 and 13. This may be more clearly seen by plotting gap scores, shown below the main profile.

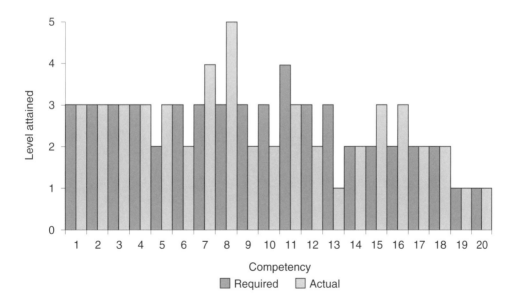

Staff competency profile.

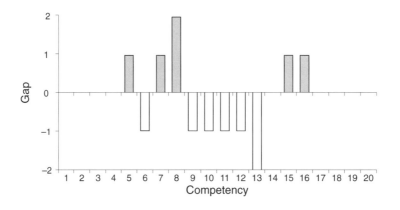

Staff competency gap profile.

The NHSIA recently provided its own set of competencies to complement *Information for Health*. These have the advantage of covering all aspects of the NHS, not just primary care, but are limited to three grades of competency.

Either competency set can be supplied to complement GPIMM. The use of the TNAMM allows the PCG(T) to audit the information training needs of all its staff and to define structured training strategies for them. The practical use of the TNAMM is illustrated opposite.

TNAMM audit screen.

TNAMM action plan screen.

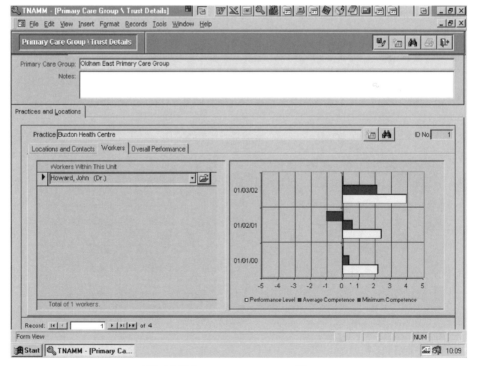

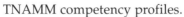

TNAMM competency profiles.

Managing the risk of computerisation

Risk management is an integral part of clinical governance and a mystery to many. However, it is an important part of managing any change process, and the computerisation of patient records is certainly a major change process.

This model associates types of risk with the IT infrastructure. Therefore it considers four types of infrastructure:

- paper-based
- single-user computerised
- network computerised
- externally linked computerised.

For the purposes of risk management we shall treat single-user and networked computerised systems as similar risks. For more information, see the original paper where this work was presented.[4]

It is possible for our purposes to map our IT infrastructure taxonomy onto our information management maturity model. This is done in the following table.

Infrastructure level	GPIMM level	Designation	Risk analysis classification
Paper-based	0	Paper-based	Paper-based
Single-user	1	Computerised	↑
↑	2	Computerised PHC team	Computerised
Multiple-user	3	Coded	
↓	4	Bespoke	↓
Externally linked	5	Paperless	Externally linked

Mapping of GPIMM classification onto risk classification.

The IT infrastructure classification represents the hardware necessary to support the level of information management activity designated within the GPIMM model.

---

[4] Gillies AC (2001) Risk management issues associated with the introduction of EHRs in primary care. *ePHI*. **1**: 1.

However, in reality many practices have an infrastructure level which exceeds that required to support their information maturity level. The risk analysis classification is associated with the hardware used, but recognises that differences between single- and multi-user systems are generally about the degree of risk rather than its nature.

In particular there has been a significant growth of risk associated with greater external connectivity arising from the advent of NHSNet. Sadly, events like the 'I love you' virus belie the reassurances regarding the integrity of the NHSNet.

From this analysis, we have classified the nature of practices in terms of their IM&T activity. The risks associated with those activities will be considered under the following headings:

- accidental damage, risks associated with actions which inadvertently lead to damage to the patient information
- deliberate damage, risks associated with actions which knowingly lead to damage to the patient information
- inherent risks, risks inherent in the use of that particular type of information system
- risks due to errors, risks arising from potential incorrect use of that particular type of information system
- risks due to ignorance, risks arising from a lack of knowledge concerning the particular type of information system, and
- opportunity risks, risks of lost opportunities arising from the nature of the type of information system used.

Thus, a matrix structure may be derived, as shown in the following table.

IT		Paper	Single	Multi-user			Linked
IM (GPIMM)		0	1	2	3	4	5
Risk	Paper		Computerised				Linked
Accidental damage							
Deliberate damage							
Inherent risks							
Risks due to errors							
Risks due to ignorance							
Opportunity risks							

Matrix structure for risk assessment.

This matrix structure will be used to consider how the risks change as IT is developed within primary healthcare.

Risk	Paper	Computerised	Linked
Accidental damage	• Records filed incorrectly and lost • Records destroyed by fire • Records destroyed by flood	• Files deleted in error • System destroyed by fire • System destroyed by flood	• System destroyed by fire • System destroyed by flood • Physical damage to communication links
Deliberate damage	• Records stolen • Records destroyed by arson	• System stolen • System destroyed by arson	• System stolen • System destroyed by arson • Deliberate damage to communication links
Inherent risks	• Records physically deteriorating due to age	• Threat from viruses • Threat from Year 2000 problem	• Threat from viruses • Threat from Year 2000 problem • Threat from external access ('hacking')
Risks due to errors	• Transcription errors • Errors in assigning Read Codes	• Data input errors • Errors due to bugs in computer system	• Data input errors • Errors due to bugs in computer system • Errors due to problems with external communication systems
Risks due to ignorance	• Failure to detect information through ignorance of record contents	• Lack of knowledge of system • Integrity problems due to failure to implement common coding standards within practice • Failure to fully implement strategies to minimise other forms of risk	• Lack of knowledge of system • Integrity problems due to failure to implement common coding standards within and without practice • Failure to fully implement strategies to minimise other forms of risk
Opportunity risks	• Difficult to get information for health promotion • Difficult to get management information • Difficult to implement coding	• Failure to reduce risk data integrity problems through electronic communications • Human and financial resources devoted to running the system	• Even greater human and financial resources devoted to running the system

Summary of risks identified within risk analysis matrix.

Accidental damage

Paper-based records are vulnerable to accidental physical damage. This can be as simple as a coffee spillage or as significant as a major fire or flood. Alternatively, paper records can be lost by incorrect filing which renders them impossible to find and therefore inaccessible. The move to computer-based systems presents analogous risks. The major incident would damage computer records as well as paper-based records. Computer files may be deleted in error, thus being lost in a similar way to a misfiled paper record.

Linked computer systems are not in themselves more vulnerable to accidental damage, but their external links may be at risk. For example, data carried on telephone wires is vulnerable to accidental damage, either airborne cables through wind damage or landlines through damage from construction work.

The significant difference is that computer systems do provide means to manage the various risks in a way that paper records are unable to do.

Deliberate damage

Deliberate physical damage affects computer-based systems in similar ways to paper-based systems. Records may be stolen, or destroyed by deliberate arson. Computer-based systems suffer the same risks. However, the intrinsic value of the computer system makes it a much higher theft risk than the paper-based equivalent. Thus, by computerising the patient records, this risk is greatly increased. It is therefore essential that strategies be adopted to reduce the risk to the patient records.

Inherent risks

Since paper-based systems are very simple compared to computer systems, inherent risks are also limited. The greatest risk inherent in a paper-based system is deterioration in paper and ink over a long period of time.

By comparison, computer systems carry much greater risk. The systems themselves carry a significant risk of mechanical breakdown, particularly in critical components such as hard disks. Since computers are dependent upon a continuous power supply, they are at risk from an interruption to the electrical power supply, either internal to the practice or externally.

In addition, computer systems face inherent risks in a number of high profile areas. Computers are threatened by viruses, programmes designed to infiltrate computer systems and then to cause damage once in place. Whilst the risk has probably been overstated, the potential damage can be severe and prevention strategies need to be adopted.

Linked systems face the additional inherent problem of 'hacking', or unauthorised external access. Any external connection to the Health Authority, Internet or

NHSNet is a potential risk. This may again be minimised by correct procedure, although, in the case of NHSNet, this may be beyond the control of the practice concerned.

Risks due to errors

The most common form of errors in paper-based systems are transcription errors. Thirty-three per cent of paper-based records may contain errors. However, fortunately, many of these are not in critical information, representing spelling errors in name and address information for example. Procedures can exacerbate this problem by placing extra steps in the data input process.

Comparable errors can be found in computer-based records. Good system design and the use of predetermined option selection from a menu as opposed to free text entry can be used to reduce error rates. This can be particularly helpful in reducing error rates in non-intuitive data such as Read Codes. However, faults in software can also introduce additional errors. Left unmanaged, this can give rise to even greater error rates, with error rates of over 50% being reported.

Similarly, in linked systems, external corruption of data transfer can introduce errors.

Risks due to ignorance

Paper-based records systems do not facilitate the detection of information within them. Therefore, users can be ignorant of the content of the records themselves. Although computers can facilitate the finding of specific information, they can also increase the risk of problems caused by ignorance.

Users of computer-based systems require knowledge of the systems themselves and ignorance of this can lead to erroneous results or a waste of resources in terms of time. Data integrity problems can be caused by ignorance of the need to implement a common coding policy across a practice. Whilst not exclusively associated with computerised practices, coding is often only implemented after computerisation. Linked practices increase this risk by requiring a common coding policy across all organisational units linked by the system.

Ignorance of strategies to reduce all forms of risk associated with computer systems in itself presents a risk, as using a computerised system without strategies for risk reduction does significantly increase risk for all the reasons outlined above.

Opportunity risks

The risk of lost opportunities within paper-based systems is very high. It is difficult to extract information for health promotion and for monitoring, evaluation and audit. It is difficult to implement a Read-coding policy. Finally, it is difficult to spot any anomalous trends that may exist within a paper-based dataset.

The opportunity risks associated with running an isolated computer system are the failure to maximise data integrity through the use of electronic communications. Further, there is an opportunity risk associated with the human and financial resources associated with running the system itself.

For linked systems, the opportunity risk associated with data integrity is reduced but the greater resources required raise that particular opportunity risk.

Case studies

These studies are based upon practices located in Greater Manchester described in a previous study by the author. However, they are assessed here from a risk management perspective and used to show differential risk at different stages of information maturity.

A paper-based practice

The practice
This practice has no computer system. It has managed with a card-based system thus far because of its small size. However, it is planned to install a system that will be linked to the FHSA. Currently, the patient records and other data are kept on card indexes. The implications of this are much greater time spent on filing and recording patient information than computerised practices that are comparable in size. More significant perhaps is the potential for error and the difficulty of spotting errors. Experience in other practices have revealed a discrepancy rate of 5–10% between paper recording systems and the FHSAs central records.

The risks
This practice represents a classic paper-based practice. It faces all the risks identified in the matrix. The practice themselves have identified the problems, and hence the plan to move to a computer-based system. However, the move to a linked computer-based system will involve many new risks that must be managed effectively.

A computerised practice: Three doctors, 5000 patients

The practice
This inner city practice had a computer system based around a single machine. Many of the characteristics of this practice arose from its inner city location.

- Due to high levels of crime in the area, it was felt that the computer could not be left in the surgery overnight. As a consequence the system was based upon a laptop machine shared by all the staff.
- The practice was characterised by a high level of patient and staff turnover.

The use of a single laptop meant that staff had limited access to the computer. The absence of formal training for staff arriving since the adoption of the system in 1991 had compounded this inexperience and led to a considerable lack of confidence amongst the administrative staff in the use of the computer. This problem was made worse by the existence of a branch surgery where all data was recorded on paper, transferred physically to the main surgery and then entered onto the computer.

These factors led to very limited use of the computer system and a dependence upon the FHSA for certain information, e.g. the FHSA supplied the list of the women to be called for cervical screening. Experience elsewhere suggests that this dependence is undesirable unless there are strong links between the doctor's own computer systems and the FHSA. This was clearly not the case here.

The system was also not used for compiling the practice report, which again causes duplication of work and introduces the possibility of data transcription errors.

The personnel interviewed, both the doctor and his staff, felt that these problems were exacerbated by poor documentation, poor training and unnecessary complexity of the computer processes.

The risks
This practice highlights how computerisation can increase risk dramatically. The most obvious example is the risk of the computer being stolen. This has in turn led to the adoption of a very limited computer-based solution, which has specific risks attached to it.

The dependency upon the FHSA has major risks associated with it in terms of data integrity. The problems with access and training increases risks due to ignorance and highlights many opportunity risks which are normally associated with paper-based systems, there are risks of information not being available for health promotion, management and monitoring.

A linked practice: One doctor, 1200 patients

The practice
This practice had a well established computer system and the doctor and his practice manager were very comfortable with the technology. Extensive use of the computer system was made for preventative medicine through screening and immunisation programs. The system used was a multi-user system with terminals

in the reception area, consulting room and practice manager's office. System maintenance and housekeeping was carried out by the practice manager, although the doctor was obviously highly computer literate. The system was used for all patient records, prescribing screening and compiling practice reports. Discussions were currently underway about direct links to the FHSA for reporting purposes. Confidentiality issues were a high priority and a mailbox system was under discussion to prevent the FHSA from having general access to the system.

The biggest problem highlighted was the transfer from manual to computer patient records. Apart from the issue of the amount of time involved, the quality of information was considered critical. Thirty three per cent of paper-based records showed inconsistencies, e.g. members of the same household were listed as living at different addresses. As a result, the input of patient data was handled by the doctor himself, in order to preserve the integrity of the data as far as possible.

The risks

This practice highlights how a well-organised practice can adopt strategies to manage and actively reduce risks. The process of computerisation was used to actively reduce the risk of data integrity errors from the original paper system. The additional risks associated with linkage are well understood and managed.

The overall effect of computerisation is that the risk to information integrity within the practice has been significantly reduced through the well managed introduction of a linked computerised system.

GRIM: a structured program for information risk management in general practice

From the analysis presented it has been stated that the overall effect of computerisation is to increase risk but to also increase the potential for that risk to be managed and reduced. The analysis can be used to identify the key elements of a General practice Risk Information Management (GRIM) program. The following table summarises the specific risks identified, their respective types together with solutions and specific actions, followed by a questionnaire designed to implement this programme within a general practice.

Specific risk	Risk type	Solution(s)	Actions
Records deleted in error	Accidental damage	Appropriate system design through appropriate dialogs and access levels	1 Audit system 2 Remedial training if required 3 Feed into procurement process
System destroyed by fire/flood	Accidental damage/ deliberate damage	Ensure adequate physical protection Ensure adequate backups of data	4 Check fire alarm systems 5 Establish and/or monitor backups Daily (incremental) Weekly (full) Monthly (remote)
System stolen	Deliberate damage	Ensure adequate physical protection Ensure adequate backups of data	6 Check intruder alarm systems 7 Establish and/or monitor backups as above
Computer viruses	Inherent	Virus protection strategy Reduce exposure risk	8 Purchase virus protection software 9 Restrict access of floppy disks and/or e-mail to the system
Data input errors	Due to errors	Appropriate system design through appropriate dialogs and access levels	10 Audit level of input errors 11 Remedial training if required 12 Audit system 13 Feed into procurement process
Errors due to bugs in system	Due to errors	Error rectification through fix or upgrade	14 Confirm system error 15 Report system error to supplier 16 Notify users of problem 17 Monitor fix by supplier
Lack of knowledge of system	Due to ignorance	Improve user knowledge of system	18 Audit user knowledge 19 Implement remedial training programme
Failure to implement common coding policy	Due to ignorance	Implement common coding policy	20 Persuade all staff to use common Read Codes 21 Train all staff in use of common Read Codes

Specific risk	Risk type	Solution(s)	Actions
Data integrity problems with external agencies	Opportunity risks	Implement external links with other agencies	22 Monitor coding for compliance to agreed policy 23 Agree communications standards with other agencies 24 Agree common coding policy with other agencies

General practice Risk Information Management (GRIM) programme.

Audit questionnaire to facilitate the implementation of the GRIM programme

Risk 1: Records deleted in error
1 a) Has an audit of the system been carried out to ensure appropriate system design through appropriate dialogs and access levels?
Yes ❑   No ❑
1 b) Has any required remedial training been carried out?
Yes ❑   No ❑ Not required ❑
1 c) Has a note been made to inform any future procurement process?
Yes ❑   No ❑ Not required ❑

Risk 2: System destroyed by fire/flood/theft
2 a) Have the fire alarms and other fire safety systems been approved by an appropriate authority?
Yes ❑   No ❑
2 b) Have the intruder alarms and other security systems been approved by an appropriate authority?
Yes ❑   No ❑
2 c) Is there a regular schedule of inspections of fire alarms and other fire safety systems?
Yes ❑   No ❑
2 d) Is there a regular schedule of inspections of security systems?
Yes ❑   No ❑

2 e) Are the following backup procedures in place?
Daily (incremental)   Yes ❑   No ❑
Weekly (full)   Yes ❑   No ❑
Monthly (remote)   Yes ❑   No ❑

Risk 3: Computer viruses

3 a) Does the organisation have a policy to prevent viruses entering the system where possible, through limits on access of floppy disks and/or e-mail to the system?
Yes ❑   No ❑

3 b) Does the organisation use adequate virus protection software?
Yes ❑   No ❑

Risk 4: Data input errors

4 a) Has an audit of the level of input errors been carried out?
Yes ❑   No ❑

4 b) If required, has a programme of remedial training been carried out?
Yes ❑   No ❑   Not required ❑

4 c) Has a note been made to inform any future procurement process?
Yes ❑   No ❑   Not required ❑

Risk 5: Errors due to bugs in system

5 a) Has a system been set up to monitor and investigate system errors?
Yes ❑   No ❑

5 b) Has a system been set up to report system errors to the supplier?
Yes ❑   No ❑

5 c) Has a system been set up to notify users of problems?
Yes ❑   No ❑

5 d) Has a system been set up to monitor fixes by the supplier?
Yes ❑   No ❑

Risk 6: Lack of knowledge of system

6 a) Has an audit been carried out to establish current levels of user knowledge?
Yes ❑   No ❑

6 b) Has any required remedial training been carried out?
Yes ❑   No ❑   Not required ❑

Risk 7: Failure to implement common coding policy

7 a) Have all staff agreed to use a common coding policy across the practice?
Yes ❑   No ❑

7 b) Have all staff been trained to use a common coding policy across the practice?
Yes ❑   No ❑

7 c) Has a monitoring procedure been introduced to validate the use of a common coding policy across the practice?
Yes ❑   No ❑

7 d) Have all staff agreed to use a common coding policy across the PCG?
Yes ❑   No ❑

7 e) Have all staff been trained to use a common coding policy across the PCG?
Yes ❑   No ❑

7 f) Has a monitoring procedure been introduced to validate the use of a common coding policy across the PCG?
Yes ❑   No ❑

Risk 8: Data integrity problems with external agencies

8 a) Have all linked organisations agreed to use a common coding policy?
Yes ❑   No ❑

8 b) Have all staff within the organisations been trained to use a common coding policy?
Yes ❑   No ❑

8 c) Has a monitoring procedure been introduced to validate the use of a common coding policy?
Yes ❑   No ❑

Conclusion to Part I

By now you may be feeling that this is the longest introduction to a book in history. However, the electronic patient record system is the foundation of any electronic disease register. Without a secure foundation, all building is wasted. By the time that you have solid information processes, well trained staff and an appreciation of the risks, then you stand a reasonable chance of implementing an electronic disease register that works.

Part Two

Fylde PCG: a case study

Chapter 4

The case study and its context

Introduction to Fylde and its PCG

Fylde covers the coastal and inland area between Blackpool and Preston in NW Lancashire. In between relatively affluent communities lie pockets of relative deprivation and as a whole the area is the 199th most deprived out of 354 English local authorities. Over a third of the population are over 55; 26% of adult men and 20% of women smoke.

The PCG board comprises a full complement of seven GPs drawn from a cross section of the nine local practices, from single handed to 5–6 doctor partnerships with branch surgeries – a total of about 38 doctors.

In common with many PCGs, Fylde identified coronary heart disease as a priority for attention, in line with the national aim to reduce deaths from circulatory disease by 40% by 2010. It is a major issue in NW Lancashire, being the cause of around 500 deaths per year.

	Age-standardised Death Rates from all circulatory disease in 1995–7 (per 100 000 people aged under 75)		
	England and Wales	North West Region	Fylde
Men	197	232	183
Women	88	107	77
Total	141	167	126

Primary Care IM&T in North West Lancashire: a GP perspective

The Fylde programme for CHD secondary prevention has been an important step in structuring disease management in the locality. The combination of payments linked to an initial audit, a requirement for a 'CHD improvement plan' and a repeat audit to determine progress has proved to be manageable for most practices.

The programme has raised issues of how data is recorded in the PCG area and aims to reward practices for following a consistent approach. The specification of Read Codes to be used and offering search criteria for use on the computer system help to provide an information structure that will answer the questions asked by the CHD audit.

The programme has now been superseded by the introduction of the NSF for coronary heart disease, which sets ambitious milestones and audit criteria and also includes primary prevention. Some of the issues around integrating the current local CHD programme into the requirements of the NSF are discussed later. The principles developed can hopefully be applied to future NSF implementations that are imminent.

The requirements of clinical governance, increased accountability and the wish to continuously improve the quality of care are important motivators for most primary care managers. Doctors and nurses are keen to demonstrate that they are providing a high quality service. As ever there is a danger that audit and data collection start to be seen as the main drivers of clinical activity rather than the real drivers, which are about patients and their problems.

For this reason every effort is made to have local data collected as a by-product of providing and documenting good clinical care, and not introduced as a separate activity.

Entering codes on the computer will improve the results of an audit report but the codes are worthless if they do not represent effective clinical activity.

It does not seem realistic to expect clinicians to record data without a clear clinical benefit. If the benefit is not apparent the data is not likely to be recorded.

This critical approach to data collection is encouraged – most clinicians do not wish to be swamped by priorities of recording data over listening to and caring for patients.

The four PCGs in NW Lancashire have been discussing the issues around collecting data at regular meetings over the last two years. In common with general practice at large we have widespread use of expensive computers within practices but no real consistency in how they are used.

The larger PCGs in NW Lancashire have been faced with rationalising the number of clinical systems in use within the PCG area, reducing it to two or three systems. This should allow quicker and easier extraction of data and offer benefits in training provision, sharing of expertise and cost savings.

The benefits of using Read Codes consistently will be more apparent as data starts to be analysed across practices and PCG areas. Savings in time and cost are expected for both the practice and PCG if raw data can be extracted from practice systems, aggregated, analysed and compared. This is the expected role of software such as MIQUEST, which is increasingly viewed as an important tool in producing health information from general practice computer systems.

In the past audits have been performed at practice level using search facilities on the practice computer system, with the results usually being transferred to paper forms which are forwarded to the health authority or MAAG.

In the future this method is likely to be superseded by the use of remote extraction of the data (with appropriate safeguards) across the NHSNet directly to the agencies requiring the data.

The vision outlined in 'Information for Health' (the NHS plan for IT implementation) is ambitious and is expected to produce an electronic health record (EHR) available to clinicians. The latest out-of-hours recommendations (2000) already specify requirements for new information flows to be established before the EHR is fully available. This has further drawn attention to the way we currently collect information about our patients and the importance of 'data quality'. General practice is building the core for the future electronic health record and attention to these issues is needed sooner rather than later.

The Read Codes if used consistently across the PCG will allow for a more centralised processing of data and make best use of the staff time and the scarce skills available.

The speed and volume of data flow now expected from general practices makes the continued use of paper records impractical and inefficient. Good clinical care in the future will require the use of computer tools and high quality data as the norm rather than an option. It will be increasingly difficult to claim to be offering high quality care without making use of the current and emerging computer technologies, especially in areas such as decision support.

As many are learning, the use of computer technology and being a caring clinician are not mutually exclusive. Problems with integrating technology into daily working patterns can usually be overcome. For some the changes needed are too much to ask and this can have a significant impact on the ability to provide comprehensive data. This needs to be tackled sympathetically on a local basis. For some it may simply be an issue of training and support but for others it may require an alternative method of collecting the data.

The recently released Amendment (No. 4) Regulations (October 2000) SI 2383 that amends paragraph 36 of Schedule 2 to the National Health Service (General Medical Services) Regulations 1992 (the terms of service) allows GPs to keep records either solely on computer or combined with paper records. There is a new requirement for this to be agreed formally with health authorities (not PCGs or PCTs) and practices may have difficulty complying if all their clinicians are not fully committed to the effective use of the clinical system.

Key components to successful data collection and coding are not only concerned with the technologies but also very much concerned with the systems developed to collect data and the involvement of the key clinicians. A lack of training and poor awareness of the issues has been the case for the majority of practices. Most GPs and practice nurses have been given limited training on the best use of their clinical computer system and are often unaware of the powerful tools they have already available. System suppliers report that the majority of requests from practices for computer system improvements are for features that are already there! Similarly PCGs may feel that bespoke systems are needed to provide the information they require rather than effective use of the systems currently being underused. This can be an expensive oversight.

To address these priority needs NWLHA has agreed to the introduction of a mentorship scheme that will provide IT support to the clinicians in primary care linked to PGEA/personal development and aimed at enhancing the use of IT in the direct care of patients. This has proved a popular approach in a number of areas in the North West – our local scheme is awaited with eager anticipation.

Some of the issues and lessons around implementing the PCG policy for CHD are included in the subsequent chapters, as are suggestions on meeting the data requirements of the NSF for CHD.

The principles outlined are equally applicable to other disease areas and, although two of the major GP systems are looked at in detail, the principles can be used with other RFA accredited GP clinical systems.

The practice manager perspective

Primary care in the National Health Service (NHS) has changed substantially in the last decade. In recent years, structural changes, most notably the introduction of primary care groups, have highlighted the need for adopting meaningful measures of quality of the primary care service.

In 1997 the UK Government began to step up its drive towards ensuring that the 'new NHS' had quality at its heart. Clinical governance was one of the central ideas in a range of proposals to modernise the NHS over a ten year period, part of a developmental programme of work. It is seen as evolutionary rather than revolutionary. The concept of clinical governance was first introduced in the NHS White Paper, entitled *The New NHS: modern, dependable.*[5] The document proposed a monitoring of clinical behaviour by a system of clinical governance triggered by a number of reported incidents in the NHS (in which questionable clinical practices continued unchecked) – press coverage was emotive and

[5] Department of Health (1997) *The New NHS: modern, dependable.* The Stationery Office, London.

hostile, raising doubts about not just isolated lapses of care but also the possibility of more systematic failings.[6]

Clearly the modernisation agenda requires the capture, generation, use and continuous monitoring of high quality information spanning two critical areas, the effectiveness of treatment and care and the clinical performance of those delivering services within the NHS.

The process of modernisation and harnessing of new technologies in healthcare also brings a requirement to equip healthcare professionals with the right motivation, skills and knowledge to deliver the agenda.

The key to using information is to balance and integrate it in an interactive process of care systems, putting it in context within the local health improvement plan, people and technology.[7]

Roper and Cutler (1998) suggest that there are three requirements for accountability of systems if they are to work effectively:[8]

- they should include a health plan and service measures that produce information that is valued by health care consumers, purchasers and providers
- there should be sufficient standardisation in measurement so that valid comparisons can be made across plans
- the measures should be amenable to efficient data collection processes in order to minimise the costs of quality measurement.

The writers also identify two types of obstacles to achieving accountability: technical and procedural, resulting in balancing the need for measuring that which is measurable and measuring that which is meaningful.

Healthcare professionals have traditionally organised their clinical communications in different ways, including:

- free text
- coded data, e.g. Read Codes
- templates facilitating structured data entry.

Historically there has been no widespread agreement about what should be recorded, and how or why. Instead, there is considerable variation in the way in which clinical information is structured and organised.

[6] Davies HT and Shields AV (1999) Public trust and accountability for clinical performance: lessons from the national press reportage of the Bristol hearing. *Journal of Evaluation in Clinical Practice*. 5(3): 335–42.

[7] Knight B (2000) Using information to support different ways of working. In: W Abbott, J Bryant and S Bullas (eds) *Current Perspectives in Health Informatics*. Health Informatics Committee, British Computer Society.

[8] Roper W and Cutler C (1998) Health plan accountability and reporting: issues and challenges. *Health Affairs*. 17: 152–5.

Variations can be categorised into two main types:

Structural
How the information is organised, e.g. free text, coded, coded and supplemented by free text etc.

Behavioural
The consistency with which the information is organised and recorded.

This has led to variation in information for individuals, professional groups and organisations over time.

The use of standard coding policies and developing models of data recording requires an evolutionary approach to ensure consistency and changes in behaviour of multi-professional groups that develop to match multi-faceted requirements over time.

It is the aim of the following sections to contribute to the quality of care by considering the processes involved in developing a framework that supports the consistent organisation and sharing of information about health and management of a given condition at a given point in time.

It is apparent that with an increasing emphasis on monitoring the quality of patient care delivered within the health service and the development of more complex forms of multi-professional working, the need for consistency in the recording and extraction of data becomes evident.

The need for education and training to support the improvement in clinical communications is essential if PCGs are to develop common frameworks for communicating information from health records to satisfy individual and organisational compliance with the delivery of quality healthcare and should be incorporated into clinical education programmes.

To be fit for purpose, any framework should be determined by clinical requirement ensuring that core clinical information is recorded during individual interventions. The time taken to access information from individual records should decrease as standard criteria for data recording will ensure the availability of core information for peer and quality improvement. It is important to note that seamless methods of extraction should not remove the clinical responsibility to validate the information and develop trust and understanding of roles and competencies across professional boundaries.

Effective communication is the essential ingredient for developing a culture conducive to quality improvement, and should be two-way, open, and designed to generate trust based on the care of the patient/client regardless of organisational structures.

Information should be assembled from systems to meet core requirements to support related processes. These processes are:

- clinical audit
- performance improvement and review
- accountability to PCG/health authority
- public health data for the monitoring of health improvement, needs assessment and service planning
- EHR to support 24 hour care provision.

The key to success is to recognise that the process should be based on team decisions, clearly identifying the necessity for commitment within teams to manage their own performance with constant monitoring and the ability to respond to the outcomes rapidly through appropriate rewards and recognition.

The next section will examine the processes involved in establishing a coding policy within a PCG to allow the measurement, monitoring, benchmarking and evaluation of service delivery, in line with national priorities and standards, whilst being responsive to local needs.

Chapter 5

Establishing agreed policies across the PCG

Introduction

The first step towards our electronic disease register is the establishment of common coding standards across the PCG.

Communication channels should be established creatively and simply to ensure inclusivity. There is no single national or international formula to describe the process of 'cracking the code', success depends on developing consensus via local, multidisciplinary teams, for specific patient/client groups. Dedicated facilitation and support is required if clinical staff are to feel included in the development of the process.

The development process begins with multidisciplinary dialogue to allow the identification and agreement on the standards to be adopted for monitoring purposes. Discussion should commence with the care the team feels should be provided for their patient/client groups. There is a need to integrate services across organisational and agency boundaries facilitating multidisciplinary liaison, streamlining the process adopted in delivering care and clarifying roles and responsibilities within teams. Healthcare professionals should feel they have been instrumental, in partnership with patients and carers, in describing appropriate care and standards of service for their patients/clients if there is to be confidence in subsequent seamless extraction, monitoring, benchmarking and evaluation of the effectiveness of treatment and care and the clinical performance of those delivering services.

Whilst the setting and monitoring of standards of care to patients provided by a PCG or Trust is the responsibility of that organisation, patient/client care is provided by more than one organisation and therefore the health organisation should ensure that all approaches toward standard setting are compatible and agreed jointly with all relevant stakeholders.

Ideally, extraction of data should be seamless, utilising the potential of technology to enable system users to access, assemble, aggregate, and analyse data held within individual patient records that are maintained through the provision of care. The reliability of information derived will depend on the consistency and completeness of the patient records. It is important that systems provide facilities to offer suitable data entry at the point of care delivery. The true benefit of electronic health records can only be delivered if the record plays an active role in the delivery of healthcare. The aim should be to work smarter, not to duplicate effort by providing information more than once. If structured data has been recorded software should enable the extraction of that data to provide information to those who require it. Health professionals should be encouraged to take ownership and harness the potential of emerging technology effectively.

It should be recognised that different practices or teams have different approaches, skills, interests and mix of patients, so any plan should facilitate and guide practices to ensure consistency of core data components, but should allow each to develop its individual response as to how a plan should be implemented within their working environments.

Any process for agreeing a common PCG coding policy should facilitate the following:

• dialogue between multidisciplinary team to determine specific selection criteria and content of the information to be extracted from individual patient records
• identification of the prevalence of particular morbidities and changes over time
• monitoring of levels and types of activities
• progress towards health gain targets for specified patient/client groups
• compliance with National Service Frameworks
• review of the achievement of expected outcomes.

The process outlined should be dynamic and capable of being reviewed and refined as necessary.

Comparison of types of measures between clinicians, practices and PCGs benchmarked against local and national data will highlight areas for investigation or action.

The NHS Executive recommends MIQUEST as a method of extracting data via queries run on primary care clinical systems.[9] However, a baseline audit could be provided by practices by their own chosen data extraction method.

---

[9] Support for the use of MIQUEST is provided by the PRIMIS project. PRIMIS is an NHS Information Authority funded project that provides training and support to local information needs.

The process

Step 1

Setting the scene

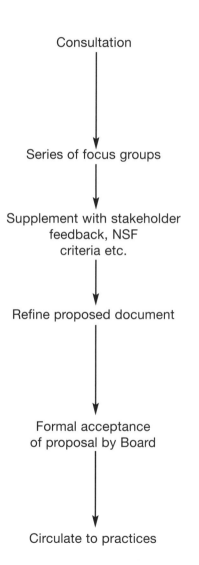

Consultation

Series of focus groups

Supplement with stakeholder
feedback, NSF
criteria etc.

Refine proposed document

Formal acceptance
of proposal by Board

Circulate to practices

Step 2
Audit/benchmarking/improvement plan

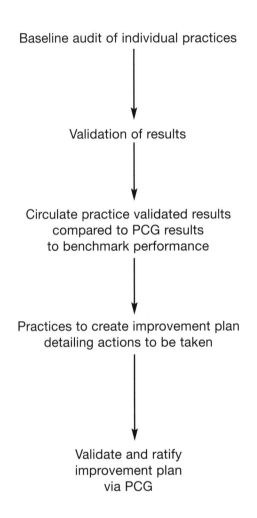

Baseline audit of individual practices

Validation of results

Circulate practice validated results
compared to PCG results
to benchmark performance

Practices to create improvement plan
detailing actions to be taken

Validate and ratify
improvement plan
via PCG

Step 3
Implement, monitor, evaluate and repeat

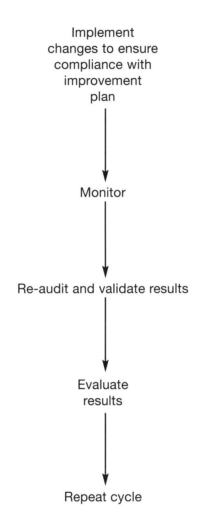

The outcome from the process

From this process an audit template was agreed, shown below:

Audit criteria	Read/BNF Code	Age range				
		<45yrs	46–60	61–75	>75	Total
1 All patients in practice						
2 All patients with CHD or atrial fibrillation	G3/G573					
From this sub-group:						
3 Patients with recorded MI	G30/G31/G32					
4 Patients with recorded coronary artery surgery	792					
5 Current smokers	137R					
6 Current non-smokers	137L					
7 Aspirin prescribed in last 2 months	BNF2.9/4.7.1					
8 Anticoagulant prescribed in last 2 months	BNF 2.8					
9 Adverse reaction to aspirin	TJ53.1					
10 Ever had cholesterol test recorded	44P					
11 Ever had LDL cholesterol > 3.1 recorded	44P6					
12 Latest LDL cholesterol recorded <3.1	44P6					
13 Lipid-lowering drugs prescribed in last 2 months	BNF 2.12					
14 Ever had blood pressure recorded	2469/246A					
15 Ever had systolic blood pressure >140 or diastolic blood pressure >85mmHg	2469/246A					
16 Latest systolic blood pressure <140 and diastolic blood pressure <85mmHG	2469/246A					
17 Nitrates and/or Digoxin prescribed in last 2 months	BNF 2.6.1/2.1					

Chapter 6

Implementing the policy

Introduction

This section is intended to build on the main process by introducing activities and associated data components, which must be supported by information assembled from, or accessed within, systems supporting integrated care activities. It will also identify factors that will need to be taken into account in proposing solutions to meet the requirements of a coding policy within a PCG.

Healthcare professionals have traditionally organised their clinical communications in a multitude of different ways. To create a robust information standard the following factors should be considered:

- appreciation of the way in which professional groups and organisations behave and communicate
- the characteristics of paper/computer-based health record systems
- standards of system design and architecture.

Coronary heart disease was the first topic chosen locally for consideration as it was the main topic in the local health improvement programme. Discussions commenced to initiate an audit of patients with pre-existing coronary heart disease and to show a reduction in the levels of the risk factors which have been proven to reduce disability and death, also to increase interventions that were proven to do likewise, e.g. the prescribing of aspirin and statins.

Steps

1 Hold a meeting to introduce the project including doctors, nurses, practice manager and administrative staff.
2 Establish training and development needs of staff to ensure that the framework will be incorporated into routine work by understanding the necessity for structural and behavioural changes in practice.
3 Identify methods of recognition and reward for participation and evidence of quality improvement against standards. Development monies could be utilised to fund the initial training and audit and recognise quality initiatives in a staged approach:

For the audit
£ per GP based on Medical Audit Advisory Group rates.

For production of a CHD Improvement Plan suggesting ways of improving key quality features
For improvements, £ per feature per GP.

Success will depend on the willingness to improve communications, both internally and externally and to share information. Protectionism needs to be replaced with openness and transparency. Most care delivery systems are done well, but there is often room for improvement and it is necessary for each generation of doctors, nurses and managers to build on existing contributions. The new agenda requires to be tackled effectively and systematically with recognition and remuneration for the work involved.

The initial audit will not simply be a measure of how well a practice performs, but also of how it records and extracts that information. The audit is just the start, and forms the foundation upon which to build.

A scheme should have four components that should be repeated at timed intervals:

- an initial audit to establish a baseline of current activity and consistency of recording standard codes
- validation of results by individual practices
- the production of an improvement plan by individual practices
- a repeat audit to determine to what extent the plan has succeeded and subsequent repeat of the whole process to ensure continuous improvement.

Completed initial audit for the practice

The completed audit for the Ash Tree House practice is shown below.

Audit criteria	Read/BNF Code	Age range				
		<45yrs	46–60	61–75	>75	Total
1 All patients in practice		6405	2280	1333	706	10724
2 All patients with CHD or atrial fibrillation	G3/G573	5	71	191	141	408
From this sub-group:						
3 Patients with recorded MI	G30/G31/G32	3	27	76	54	160
4 Patients with recorded coronary artery surgery	792	2	15	39	8	64
5 Current smokers	137R	1	17	25	11	54
6 Current non-smokers	137L	3	53	163	126	345
7 Aspirin prescribed in last 2 months	BNF2.9/4.7.1			124	87	211
8 Anticoagulant prescribed in last 2 months	BNF 2.8	1	7	31	11	50
9 Adverse reaction to aspirin	TJ53.1					
10 Ever had cholesterol test recorded	44P	4	66	186		256
11 Ever had LDL cholesterol > 3.1 recorded	44P6	0	14	44		58
12 Latest LDL cholesterol recorded <3.1	44P6	2	13	21		36
13 Lipid-lowering drugs prescribed in last 2 months	BNF 2.12	3	44	115	24	186
14 Ever had blood pressure recorded	2469/246A	5	71	191	140	407
15 Ever had systolic blood pressure >140 or diastolic blood pressure >85mmHg	2469/246A	3	67	187	140	397

Cont.

Audit criteria	Read/BNF Code	Age range				
		<45yrs	46–60	61–75	>75	Total
16 Latest systolic blood pressure <140 and diastolic blood pressure <85mmHG	2469/246A	5	21	52	28	106
17 Nitrates and/or Digoxin prescribed in last 2 months	BNF 2.6.1/2.1	2	26	96	106	230

Improvement plan

Practices will need to provide information regarding their populations, to recognise specific target groups of patients, describe their current care delivery, including which staff perform which tasks, identify areas they feel they need to address and how each of these areas will be addressed, e.g:

- Which staff will do the work?
- What extra time will this take?
- What additional administration will be needed?
- Will the tasks be undertaken with formal clinics or opportunistically?
- How will the information be recorded and how will the practice ensure that the information is accurately and consistently coded?
- What systems of recall will be developed?
- Which guidelines or frameworks will be used?

A meeting should be held to demonstrate anonymously the results of the initial audit, to give people an idea of how their practice is currently performing compared to others in the locality. Specific, individual results should be provided for individual practice use.

	Read/BNF Code	Age range				
Fylde PCG Initial Audit – Average %		<45yrs	46–60	61–75	>75	Total
1 All patients with CHD or atrial fibrillation	G3/G573	0.1%	2.7%	12.9%	18.3%	4.9%
From this sub-group:						
2 Current smokers	137R	39%	19.6%	10.5%	5.5%	9.8%
3 Current non-smokers	137L	42.3%	59.5%	72.2%	66.5%	68.3%
4 Aspirin prescribed in last 2 months	BNF2.9/4.7.1			60.2%	55.7%	58.2%
5 Ever had cholesterol test recorded	44P	51.8%	66.4%	63.6%		63.7%
6 Ever had LDL cholesterol > 3.1 recorded	44P6	5.6%	12.5%	13.3%		12.7%
7 Latest LDL cholesterol recorded <3.1	44P6	7.5%	12.6%	12.6%		12.9%
8 Ever had blood pressure recorded	2469/246A	85.7%	92.8%	89.2%	82.1%	86.4%
9 Ever had systolic blood pressure >140 or diastolic blood pressure >85mmHg	2469/246A	41.6%	61.5%	70.8%	67.2%	67.6%
10 Latest systolic blood pressure <140 and diastolic blood pressure <85mmHG	2469/246A	68.2%	43.7%	40.7%	32.8%	38.3%

Completed audit for Ash Tree House practice as percentage of practice population.

Aims of the plan

To recognise patients with pre-existing CHD as a percentage of practice population (G3) and to show a reduction in the levels of those risk factors where they have been proven to reduce disability and death, and an increase in treatments proven to do likewise.

The risk factors specified:

• smoking
• hypercholesterolaemia
• uncontrolled hypertension.

The treatment specified will be aspirin or other anticoagulant therapy.

To provide accurate and comparable computer-coded information regarding the treatment of patients with CHD.[10]

The ways that a practice will make improvements will vary from practice to practice so here are a few suggestions:

- a disease management framework which satisfies national service framework criteria and local health need requirements
- register of coded disease topic, e.g. G3
- standardisation of risk factor coding, e.g. ex-smoker, heavy smoker, aspirin prophylaxis (to include those patients who purchase their prescriptions over the counter from a pharmacist)
- use of electronic laboratory links for comparable coding and sharing of cholesterol results across primary and secondary care interfaces.

The NSF for coronary heart disease was published after the Fylde PCG initial CHD plan and specifies additional priorities and primary prevention. The purpose of the section is to demonstrate the stages of development to help structure clinical information. It is intended primarily to help understand the evolutionary nature of the processes involved.

---

[10] Hardwick SA and Mechan J (2000) How Fylde PCG put practices at the heart of its CHD plan. *Vision Doctor Supplement* (September). Reed Healthcare Publishing, Sutton.

Chapter 7

Implementing the policy in an In Practice VISION practice

The practice: Ash Tree House Surgery

The practice is situated in the old market town of Kirkham, mid-way between Blackpool and Preston, providing services to residents of rural Fylde in Lancashire.

The practice operates from a Grade II listed building with a list size of 10 674. The main surgery operates on four levels with access to all floors by lift and stairs. The practice also provides services, including dispensing, at the branch surgery at Weeton Army Camp.

The practice of six partners employs 20 staff directly, 14 attached staff and six professionals allied to medicine (counsellor, clinical psychologist, physiotherapist, chiropodist, dietician and radiographer).

The practice has the following age-sex profile:

Age	Male	Female	Total
0–4	323	368	691
5–14	707	731	1438
15–24	587	616	1203
25–34	707	822	1531
35–44	720	810	1530
45–64	1389	1379	2768
65–74	365	465	830
75–84	212	324	536
85+	36	111	147
Total	**5048**	**5626**	**10674**

The practice began planning for computerisation in 1986 and commenced in 1988 by constructing their own database from a manual age/sex register to ensure accuracy. Since 1989 the computers have been used in consultation by all clinicians and since 1993 the attached staff of district nurses and health visitors have had input to patient electronic health records.

The system: VISION

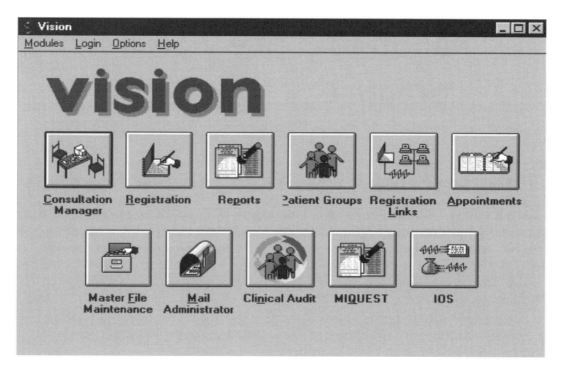

The most comprehensive method of ensuring coding compliance within VISION is to create a guideline with selected Read Codes attached behind buttons or picklists and this is described later in this section. It is also important to understand the spectrum of data entry methods available to users and to demonstrate standardised data recording and extraction whilst ensuring individuals are able to choose the method most appropriate to their own requirements for data entry.

Data is mostly entered and stored within Consultation Manager using terms from the Read dictionary. The entry is made either on a relevant screen, e.g. Blood

Pressure Add, for example, from within a Management Plan which lists suitable entries in a category, seamlessly attaching a Read Code; or to save searching around for the correct screen, you can go straight ahead and type a Read term using one of the shortcut Read entry methods. The VISION system will then place the record in the relevant structured data area (SDA), e.g. Blood Pressure.

The Read dictionary

Records on VISION are entered and stored as Read terms. Some screens already have a limited choice of relevant Read terms to choose from. A sub-set of the Read dictionary can also be created as a practice formulary, consisting of the practice's preferred Read descriptions which should be aligned to organisational coding requirements to ensure consistency of data recording and extraction.

How to enter a Read Code is explained later in this section. First, an explanation about how the Read dictionary is structured.

The Read dictionary can be accessed either using keywords (Read's or your own), or by code. It is a hierarchical structure consisting of five levels of codes, giving more detail as you go down.

The concept of keywords

Many terms can be selected from the Read dictionary by entering a keyword.

- Keywords are not simply parts of the Read term, but have been specifically attached to the Read term when the Read dictionary was designed, for example, IHD is the keyword to find ischaemic heart disease codes.
- Some Read terms have no keywords. These terms cannot be found by a keyword search, but can only be selected from the code hierarchy. G3 ... is the code for IHD – ischaemic heart disease.
- Ensure that all Read terms in your practice formulary have at least one keyword attached.
- Use a simple but effective keyword system which everybody in the practice is aware of and understands.

Read Codes have five characters. All codes begin with one of the following characters 0–9 A–Z, each being a different category of the description.

0	Occupations	G	Circulatory system diseases
1	History / symptoms	H	Respiratory system diseases
2	Examination / signs	J	Digestive system diseases
3	Diagnostic procedures	K	Genitourinary system diseases
4	Laboratory procedures	L	Complications of pregnancy, childbirth and puerperium
5	Radiology / physics in medicine		
6	Preventative procedures	M	Skin and subcutaneous tissue diseases
7	Operations, procedures, sites	N	Musculoskeletal and connective tissue diseases
8	Other therapeutic procedures		
9	Administration	P	Congenital anomalies
A	Infectious and parasitic diseases	Q	Perinatal conditions
B	Neoplasms	R	[D] Symptoms, signs and ill-defined conditions
C	Endocrine / nutritional / metabolic / immunity disorders		
		S	Injury and poisoning
D	Diseases of blood and blood forming organs	T	Causes of injury and poisoning
		U	[X] External causes of morbidity and mortality
E	Mental disorders		
F	Nervous system and sense organ diseases	Z	Unspecified conditions

Find and use the correct Read term

To find the correct Read term:

1 Decide which chapter the code is under, and determine level in hierarchy accordingly. Pick the correct type to ensure reliable output – Chapter 1 is History and symptoms, where the systems chapters A–Z cover diagnoses.
2 Set up and maintain a Read Formulary with practice-specific contents to ensure ease and consistency of data entry across the whole practice team.
3 If Read codes are known, they can be entered on the History screen by preceding the code with a #, e.g. #G3 to enter ischaemic heart disease.

The following are the quick ways of selecting a Read term, by displaying a *Read Term Add* screen on the Patient Record.

When you have the Patient Record displayed, and a consultation started:

1 Start typing straightaway (for this to happen, you need to make sure that Pop-up Read Term Dialogue is checked in Consultation – Options – Setup – Patient Record).

This displays a Read Term Add window.

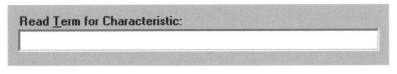

In the Read Term Add window:
- select by keyword – either type in one or two partial keywords in the Read term keywords as suggested later in this section
- select by code (hierarchy) – or if you know the Read Code, type # then the code, e.g. #G for circulatory system.

2   Press the Return key to display a Read term which matches your entry. The cursor stays in the Read Term for Characteristic window.
3   Use the down arrow key ↓ to get the next term that matches the description you want. If you cannot find what you want, press <F3> to reach the back Read Dictionary screen. The keyword will be remembered in Keyword, and a list of relevant descriptions are displayed.
4   Look at the hierarchical list (it remembers what you typed in) and select the description you want by double clicking on it.
5   Put this term in the Formulary if it is used regularly.

If you right mouse click at the Read Dictionary screen, you can see the keyword, if any, of the code that is currently highlighted.

Medical acronyms used for Read selection:

Read Code	Acronym	Term	In Read already
G3...13	IHD	IHD – Ischaemic heart disease	Yes
G573.00	AF	Atrial fibrillation and flutter	Yes

The Patient Record View

The Patient Record View has been designed to allow flexible viewing and recording of patient data from a single screen. The layout of the Patient Record View can be customised to suit the individual user.

This is how the Patient Record looks for a patient whose consultation has started, but for which no new data has been added.

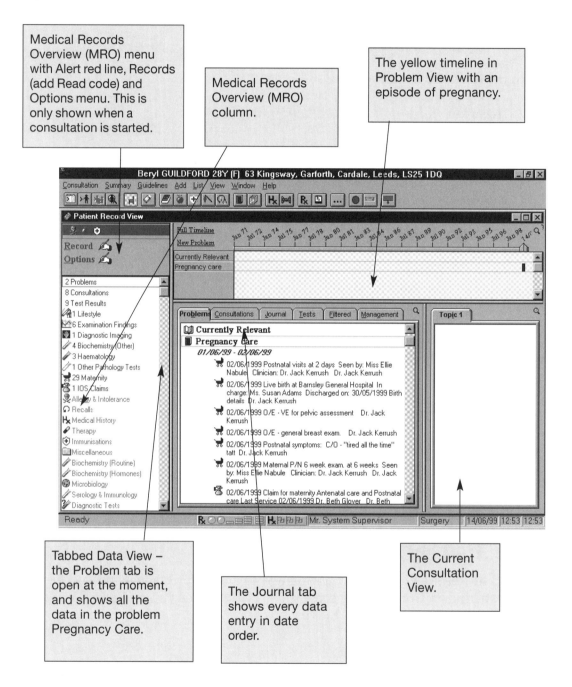

Medical Records Overview (MRO) menu with Alert red line, Records (add Read code) and Options menu. This is only shown when a consultation is started.

Medical Records Overview (MRO) column.

The yellow timeline in Problem View with an episode of pregnancy.

Tabbed Data View – the Problem tab is open at the moment, and shows all the data in the problem Pregnancy Care.

The Journal tab shows every data entry in date order.

The Current Consultation View.

Journal tab

The Journal tab on Patient Record View lists all the data for the patient in reverse date order.

Management tab

The Management tab displays guidelines – either Management Plans, which are grid-format guidelines helping data entry, or local or Prodigy guidelines. Right mouse click on a line on the MRO column and select Management Plan.

Other sorts of guidelines are Prodigy guidelines, issued centrally by the Government, or local guidelines – those you have created yourself or imported.

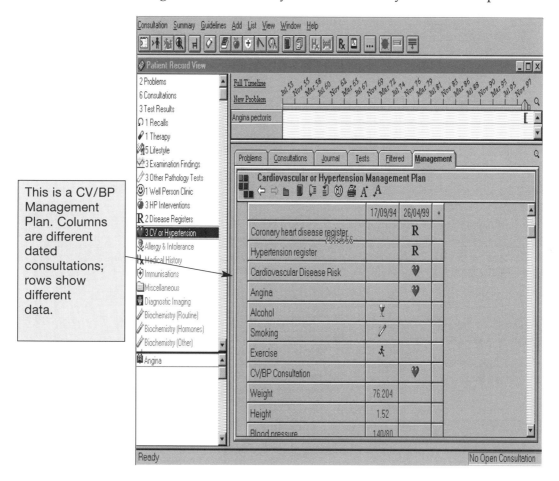

This is a CV/BP Management Plan. Columns are different dated consultations; rows show different data.

Data entry from the Patient Record View

The Patient Record View offers multiple ways of adding new data in the current consultation. There is no right or wrong way, and quite often different methods are just a matter of personal preference. The easiest is probably to right mouse click on a line on the MRO column and select either Summary Form or Management Plan, though some single entries are more straightforward using the Add menu.

The following methods for entering data are meant as a general guide – each user should decide individually which method suits best.

Data entry via the Toolbar

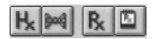

History, Referral, Acute Therapy, Repeat Therapy.

You can directly access a Data Add screen by clicking on one of these icons.

History Add	?

Event Date: 22 January 1998
Clinician: Dr. Jack Kensch
☐ Private
☒ In Practice

Head Term for Characteristic:

Comment:

Another
OK
Cancel

Type of Characteristic: Diagnosis
Episode Type: Other
Priority: 3

Help

End Date:

> The Medical History screen can be used for any data entry using the Read dictionary. The system will offer to place the record in the structured data area that is relevant, e.g. if you enter Asthma, it is placed in the Asthma area; if you enter C/O cough, it stays as a general history entry.

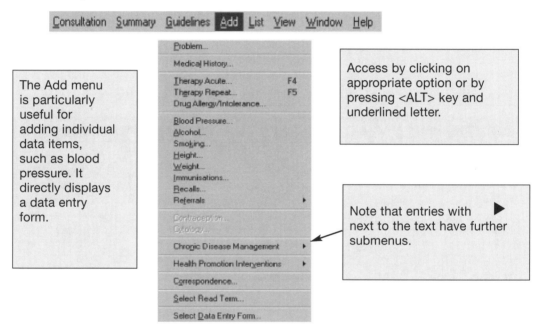

Chronic Disease Registers, Health Promotion, Immunisations, Prevention Display, Select Summary Form.

Access one of these summary and tabbed forms from their icons on the toolbar, then use the right mouse menu to add new data. Especially useful for multiple related entries.

Data entry via the Menu bar

Access the Add menu by pressing the <ALT> key and then the letter A. The individual entries on the menu can then be selected by pressing the underlined letter.

Data entry via the Summary Form menu on the MRO

Right mouse clicking on most lines on the Medical Records Overview column will let you choose Summary Form. This displays the appropriate summary form, some of which are tabbed. You can then use the right mouse menu to add data.

This is the summary form for Examination Findings, or Physiological Measurements. Point to Examination Findings on MRO, right-mouse click, then select Summary Form.

To make a new entry, point to prompt, e.g. BP, right-mouse click, then left-mouse, click on Add.

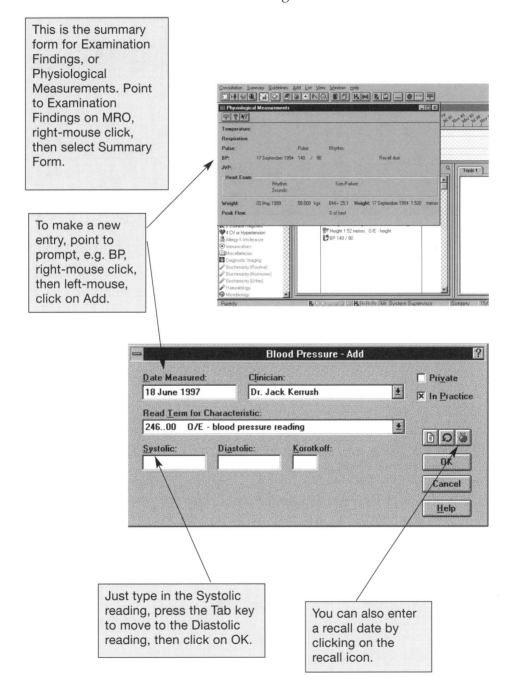

Just type in the Systolic reading, press the Tab key to move to the Diastolic reading, then click on OK.

You can also enter a recall date by clicking on the recall icon.

Data entry by just starting to type a keyword or Read Code for any clinical entry

Providing the option for Popup Read Term Dialogue is enabled on the Setup screen for Consultation Manager, pressing any key on the keyboard will invoke the Read Term Dialogue box.

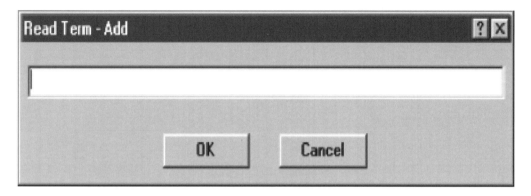

In summary when entering Read Codes you can:

- enter a keyword for the required entry and press Enter – the first matching entry will be displayed
- if the displayed entry is the correct one, click on the OK button or press Enter twice to accept the entry
- if the displayed entry is not correct, double click on it or press the F3 function key to display the Read Dictionary screen. Select the appropriate entry from there
- the most appropriate screen for the selected Read term will be displayed. In most cases this will be the Medical History screen. Depending on the selected Read term a 'structured data area', i.e. a special data entry screen relevant for that Read term, may be displayed for data entry
- if the Read Code is known, this can be entered directly by prefixing the code with a # sign, e.g. # G3 for Ischaemic Heart Disease. Note that after entering and accepting a Read term, you may well:
  - trigger a Prodigy guideline, or one of your local guidelines, if that Read term acts as a trigger
  - create a new problem, or open an existing problem again, if the Read term is a triggering Read term for a guideline and the existing problem has the same mnemonic as the triggered guideline.

Management Plans

The Management tab of the Patient Record View can be used either to display Management Plans (part of the VISION system, or locally created by yourself), or to display Prodigy guidelines, especially those triggered from the Read term entered.

From the left-hand MRO column of the Patient Record View screen, you can point to one of the following lines, click with the right mouse and choose Management Plan as an alternative to Summary Form:

• Lifestyle, Examination Findings, Pathology Tests and X-ray Results, Disease Registers, Asthma, Immunisations, New Registration Exam, Well Person Clinic, Health Promotion Interventions, Diabetes, CV or Hypertension, Elderly, Epilepsy

Right-mouse click on an MRO line and select Management Plan.

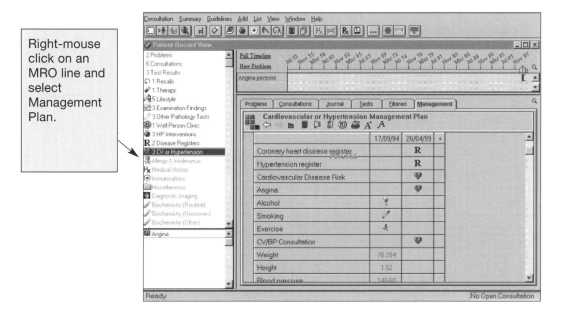

CV/Hypertension Management Plan.

These Management Plans are also called Data Snapshot cards. They are types of guidelines, mostly in grid format, displaying a selected portion of the patient record. Their advantage is that they can show the user the episodes of data, especially useful for such categories as test results.

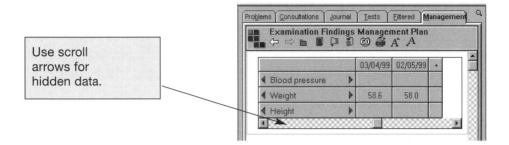

If you right mouse click on one of the rows in the left-hand column, other than the header row, you have additional options:

- Graph – To display a graph of data on that row, if plottable as a graph
- Add – To make a new entry for that date.

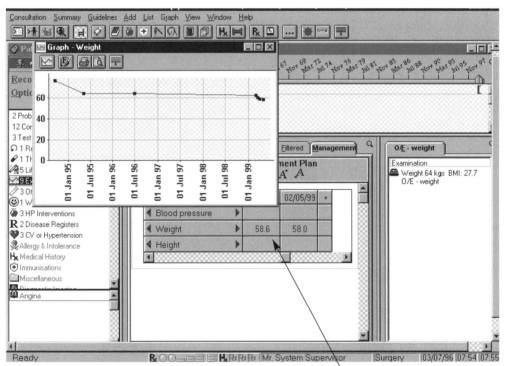

Weight Graph: Examination Findings Management Plan.

Right-mouse click on a line with numerical entries, e.g. weight, BP, Hb, and select Graph.

Guidelines

The concept of guidelines in VISION encompasses three major areas:

Patient Reports – some reports come with the VISION system and others are user definable. Reports filter existing patient data under different criteria and display specific data according to age and sex. Patient reports can be printed for individual patients or groups of patients.

Data entry screens – both Prodigy and user definable (local) guidelines, as well as displaying existing patient data filtered under different criteria, can also contain data entry buttons or icons, lists of drugs and Read descriptions and buttons or icons to launch external applications.

Disease and prescribing protocols – Prodigy guidelines can use the full range of features available which in addition to the ones already mentioned above can also include prescribing regimes, printable patient information and on-line pictures and video clips. These screens can be triggered by one or more Read Codes, i.e. when a history entry is made with a triggering Read Code or a code further down the same hierarchy as the triggering Read Code, the guideline will be offered for display. You can define your own local guidelines or import guidelines. The following guideline was downloaded from the InPS web site and imported. Acknowledgement goes to Bury North Primary Care Group for the creation of this guideline which complies with the NSF for coronary heart disease.

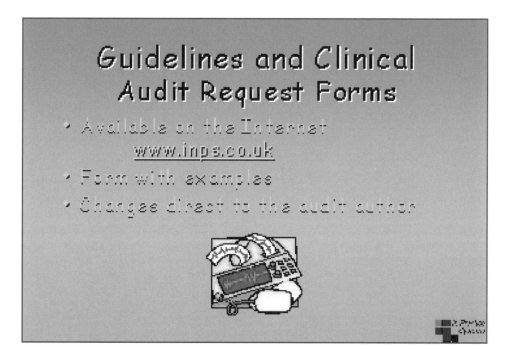

Albert ALLEN 78Y (M) 27 Marston Road, Teddington, Middx, TW11 8AH

Consultation   Summary   Guidelines   Add   List   View   Window   Help

Coronary Heart Disease Guidelines - 1.0 (BNPCG)

Coronary Heart Disease Guidelines - 1.0 (BNPCG)

Background

Significant CHD and OAD events
16/09/2000 Left ventricular failure   Dr. A. Demo
16/09/2000 Angina pectoris   Dr. A. Demo
16/09/2000 Ischaemic heart disease   Dr. A. Demo
To enter diagnosis - press here

CHD monitoring records
16/09/2000 Cardiac disease monitoring   Dr. A. Demo
Previous records - press here

Relevant Investigations
18/10/1999 ECG - general Normal Dr. Alison Cool
All ECG exercise Records - No data available.
16/09/2000 Echocardiogram Dr. A. Demo
All Coronary angiogram Records - No data available.
To enter relevant investigation - press here

Next Recall

Acute otit
Middle ear flui
Angina
Asthma
Asthma - Children under 5
Chest Infections

Tell your doctor if you are taking any other medication.
BP 120 / 80 O/E - BP reading

Ready   Mr. System Supervisor   Go Home   16/09/00 16:13 16:22

Coronary Heart Disease Guidelines - 1.0 (BNPCG)

Background

Significant CHD and OAD events

16/09/2000 Left ventricular failure   Dr. A. Demo
16/09/2000 Angina pectoris   Dr. A. Demo
16/09/2000 Ischaemic heart disease   Dr. A. Demo
To enter diagnosis - press here

CHD monitoring records

16/09/2000 Cardiac disease monitoring   Dr. A. Demo
Previous records - press here

Relevant Investigations

18/10/1999 ECG - general Normal Dr. Alison Cool
All ECG exercise Records - No data available.
16/09/2000 Echocardiogram Dr. A. Demo
All Coronary angiogram Records - No data available.
To enter relevant investigation - press here

Next Recall

16/09/1999 Recall on 16/09/2000 for Cardiac disease monitoring with Dr. A. Demo

----

Risk Factor Recording

Other relevant conditions - Hypertension & Diabetes

06/07/1993 Essential hypertension   Dr. Edna Frosty
22/01/1997 Diabetes mellitus   Dr. Edna Frosty
22/01/1997 Diabetes mellitus   Dr. Edna Frosty
To enter diagnosis - press here

Lifestyle factors

	22/01/1999	26/08/1999	26/08/1999 31/08/1999	31/08/1999	02/12/1999	16/09/2000	+
◀ Smoking ▶		🖉	🖉	🖉	🖉		
◀ Alcohol ▶			⚲				
◀ Exercise ▶	🏃						
◀ Diet ▶						🍽	

Physiological & Biochemical factors

	26/08/1999	26/08/1999	29/09/1999	26/10/1999	02/12/1999	10/08/2000	+
◀ BP (<140/85 ▶	120/80	120/80	150/95	150/90	140/80	120/80	
◀ BMI (M<25:F ▶							
◀ TC (<5.0) ▶							

◀ ▶

Interventions
    Patient Education
    Medication
        Aspirin - all patients
           16/09/2000 ASPIRIN disp tab 75mg Supply: (100) tablet(s) 1 EVERY DAY Dr. A. Demo
           TO PRESCRIBE
           CONTRA-INDICATIONS
        Beta-blockers - all patients especially after MI
           No data recorded
           TO PRESCRIBE
           CONTRA-INDICATIONS

References
    1 The National Service Framework - Coronary Heart Disease (2000) - www.doh.gov.uk/nsf/coronary.htm

The sample data illustrates the target population and the trigger clinical entry that determines membership of that group. The group can be then used to publish Post-it notes on individual screens to enable appropriate interventions. The audit should be re-run on a monthly basis to monitor compliance with the local health improvement plan and NSF criteria, demonstrating improvement in healthcare.

Data analysis

The data produced by running these reports can be read as tables, or can be exported to a package such as Excel, to produce graphs of the type shown in Part 1.

A sample graph of the type produced at Ash Tree House Surgery is shown opposite.

Further details of how to export your data from VISION and how to manipulate it in Excel are given in Gillies A (2001) *Excel for Clinical Governance*. Radcliffe Medical Press, Oxford.

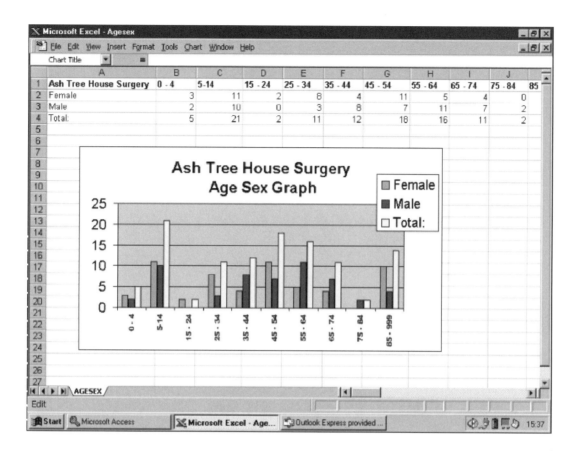

		A	B	C	D	E	F	G	H	I	J	
			0 - 4	5-14	15 - 24	25 - 34	35 - 44	45 - 54	55 - 64	65 - 74	75 - 84	85
1	Ash Tree House Surgery											
2	Female		3	11	2	8	4	11	5	4	0	
3	Male		2	10	0	3	8	7	11	7	2	
4	Total:		5	21	2	11	12	18	16	11	2	

Implementing the CHD policy in an EMIS practice

The practice: Holland House Surgery

The practice is long established in the coastal town of Lytham and has five full-time partners, three practice nurses, a dedicated team of reception and clerical staff and a complement of attached staff working in the district.

The practice covers a broad area along a coastal strip, a mostly urban population but also covering the more rural areas inland. Working from two sites the EMIS system is linked to both surgeries and recently access to NHSNet has been provided from both sites. This provides great flexibility in access to the electronic record and electronic communications.

The surgery receives all laboratory results electronically including x-rays and cervical cytology and these are filed directly in to the patient records and therefore readily available in templates etc.

All hospital letters received are scanned and converted to text using optical character recognition (OCR) for inclusion into the patient records. Paper records are still maintained and are being systematically summarised into an electronic form. The practice will be seeking approval to hold electronic records under the new GP terms of service (NHS GMS Amendment (No.4) Regulations 2000 – SI 2383) – see also www.doh.gov.uk/gpepr.

As the doctors still provide the out-of-hours cover there is also access to the system from external sites.

Computer use in the surgery has progressed from a single machine in the late 1980s to the current Windows NT network using predominantly PCs. While not being a 'paperless' practice, ways of working have changed significantly. Clinicians all now consult using the EMIS system within consultations and all contacts relating to patients are recorded on the system.

Many developments have been made as the result of suggestions from the wider practice team. A number of the team are familiar with the concepts of Read Codes and are able to summarise and update records to produce high levels of data quality.

Funding from the health authority has supported local training for the wider team. The role of 'clinical coding' within the practice is growing in importance and makes life a lot easier for the clinicians who are not able to undertake the task of summarising and maintaining electronic records on top of their usual commitments.

The need to fulfil the requirements of the Data Protection Act and the Caldicott recommendations is considered during any development. Access to patient records is intended to be on a 'need to know' basis and this is respected as far as it can be within the limits of the software.

The clinicians record details of consultations and refer to various aspects of the electronic record with updating prescription lists and episode management, e.g. re-categorising of problems on the record from active to past. All prescribing is via the computer system and any handwritten scripts are recorded. Templates are used as a way of ensuring consistency of coding within disease areas.

Each consultation record has a code attached by the clinician to represent the diagnosis or symptom under consideration. This code can be collected from the existing list for that patient – for future consultations for the same problem the records are much more effective and allow rapid access to previous entries. Consistency in coding is a key issue where many alternative codes are available.

Opportunities to use electronic methods within the practice are always given critical consideration before being introduced on the basis of 'the tool must do the job'. Past implementation of Information Technology in the NHS has not always been successful. The introduction of computer technology brings with it a need for people to change the way they work and a requirement for training. The benefits of the change need to be clearly defined and worthwhile before committing time and effort.

From experience, the early adoption of a poorly conceived electronic system can place a strain on time and resources and can easily increase rather than decrease workload without providing any significant benefit for patients.

The Practice Computer System: EMIS: version 5 running LV2/Version 5.1 (2000/1)

Some familiarity with the use of the system is assumed and reference to the EMIS manuals provided with the system is recommended.

The EMIS main menu screen.

N.B. Codes and system configuration may change as the system is developed. If some of the menu items do not appear or are 'greyed-out' when using the system request appropriate user access from your practice system administrator. This is usually the person who designates each staff member to a user 'level' on the system.

Integrating policy into the computer system

When any new clinical policy arrives in the practice it usually arrives as a wad of paper. How is it best to translate the requirements of the policy so that it can be integrated into the clinical computer system and therefore available to the clinicians in their daily work?

First, some comments on the practicalities of clinical coding in general practice.

A data capture process – have you got one?

Enormous volumes of data and information pass through every general practice. The future promises electronic records for the NHS but until then most of us will be dealing with large volumes of paper.

A robust process for the collection of data is fundamental to generating worthwhile information. It is going to be a major part of activity in primary care in the future and so resources need to be provided for data to be collected effectively. This means having staff available and trained in the use of the clinical computer system, able to summarise and code records and use the systems as they continually evolve. The commitment and training of all the clinicians are key factors in achieving a worthwhile result.

This data collection process in the practice underpins any effort to implement and monitor a clinical policy.

A systematic 'data flow' analysis can chart the arrival, generation, modification and movement of information around and out of the practice and can identify opportunities for data to be collected and also spot where important data is likely to be missed. It can be a worthwhile exercise uncovering a surprising complexity.

It can also raise the issue of whether some processes can be simplified or rationalised and how the practice computer system could be used to better effect.

Ways to improve information availability in a practice include:

- note summarisation and data entry from paper to computer (by specially trained staff members)
- continuous pruning and updating of prescription lists
- highlighting and coding details from hospital letters and discharge summaries
- scanning of letters using OCR software or as image files
- updating and correcting records during consultations with patients
- information recorded for out of hours and home visits
- clinical templates to speed and control data entry.

Audits of data collection and data quality

The stated aims of the Fylde CHD programme have been to demonstrate an improvement in outcomes by using an audit process.

- An initial audit – run through the EMIS system.
- The setting of targets.

A repeat audit to demonstrate a positive change

Fylde PCG has eased this process by specifying the Read/EMIS codes and the audit criteria to be included. This should help with the consistency of coding and also limit the amount of extra work required at practice level to decide on codes.

The PCG has not included a matching template structure for data capture in this first program, leaving this to individual practices. A single template solution is not always possible across a variety of clinical computer systems. Where a small number of systems are in use, the provision of a ready-made template can save time for practices and further improve data quality.

Each practice and indeed each clinician has the flexibility to use the EMIS clinical system to suit individual preferences. Within a single practice it is possible for clinicians to structure their own methods of data input and audit by setting up their own templates and audit searches. Where a practice has a number of IT literate clinicians able to adapt the system, this approach is perfectly possible and the flexibility it offers is one of the strengths of using a computer system. As long as the codes used are consistent with the PCG policy and the data is of good quality it should not create a problem. This method is in use within our own practice.

While this approach is flexible it is an obvious duplication of work and if not done consistently it would create problems – it would not suit every practice. Many practices therefore decide to restrict any modification of the computer set up to a small number of individuals – this is usually a wise decision and will avoid the inevitable accumulation of half-baked or incomplete templates, searches and audits.

The work of structuring the computer system, e.g. designing templates, to gather specific data is often viewed as 'non-clinical', repetitive and uninteresting. In most practices the work will be left to a single member of staff who has the required interest and skills. This does not have to be a clinician and the work can be delegated as long as the clinical issues are well understood and the new system is efficient in the use of clinical time.

A single data collection system may not suit everyone's way of working and sometimes adaptations will be required. An example might be to use a number of smaller templates rather than one large template for CHD data input. Templates for use by a practice nurse can be structured differently to that used by a doctor – again this is feasible as long as the codes used are consistent. Most prefer to 'keep it simple' and a single and often large template is often the preferred solution.

Clinical computer systems are not transparent in their structure and colleagues will not automatically understand the new structure available to them.

It is important to spread the word, showing how to access templates etc. so that all the relevant team members are able to use the new system. This training aspect is crucial, although often overlooked. Locums and new staff members will need to be included too.

It is worthwhile to:

• outline the nature and aims of the clinical policy
• explain how the EMIS system has been changed to achieve the outcomes
• encourage feedback if the chosen structure creates problems
• know the EMIS coding structure and where to find the codes.

When selecting codes in audits and searches using EMIS, a selection will be offered and it is therefore easy to miss where a code fits into the greater structure. It is not essential to understand the Read Code hierarchy in order to build audits and searches but it can be helpful in avoiding Codes from an inappropriate section.

EMIS uses the standard Read Codes and most current systems will use the '5-Byte' codes. If you are unsure of which version you are using then check with the supplier as the older '4-Byte' version of the codes are not the same. The 5-Byte code for IHD is G3, whereas the 4-Byte code is G4 – an obvious source of confusion!

Anyone wishing to become familiar with the Read Code structure as it appears in EMIS can do so by browsing the hierarchy to see how it branches off and how the codes develop and link.

This can be done by following the main menu to

DT: Dictionaries and Templates
C: Codes, Templates and Protocols
B: Read Classification

Navigating up and down the hierarchy can be done by following the instructions on screen.

What does 'MNL' mean at the side of some codes? These refer to whether the code has an associated entry in Mentor: M, Prodigy: N (for node), Patient information leaflet: L.

```
Classifications                                                    [ ]

A  Access Screen                          B  Read Classification
E  Edit Access Screen/Forms/Templates     S  Create more synonyms
C  Clinical Protocols                     M  Advanced Code Management
F  Code Abbreviation


   NHS Clinical Terms:
   Crown copyright data reproduced by permission of the Controller of
   Her Majesty's Stationary Office








   Your read code version is 5.200009.(6)

   Select Option :
```

Tidying up coding inconsistencies

The implementation of a coding policy could well uncover past inconsistency in the use of codes, patchy recording of data etc.

The practice may have used codes incorrectly in the past or have used their own 'in-house codes' not realising that a Read Code already existed. This could be a greater problem in some practices. Some familiarity with the local use of codes will help. It is possible to use the system to replace one code by another.

In-house codes can be converted to the appropriate Read Code. Inconsistent or duplicate codes in patient records can be found by searches, adding the accepted code (with the same date as the original) and then removing the erroneous code.

It may be necessary to monitor the subsequent use of unfavoured codes to prevent the bad habits recurring. Searches for such codes can be repeated periodically to spot their continued use and to target the need for training of those still entering them or the modification of a template still containing the code.

For code management from the main menu:

DT: Dictionaries and Templates
C: Codes, Templates and Protocols
M: Advanced Code Management.

Here will be found a further menu offering a series of fundamental alterations to the coding structure and linkages.

Option H allows conversion of one code to another.

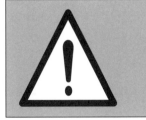

As this can have significant implications on the availability and use of the codes for all users, code changes should only be made after careful consideration and following training on use of the system for this purpose, particularly when using the 'batch data' conversion methods.

Setting up the EMIS system for the Fylde CHD programme

This is a simple method applying to a current EMIS system (2000). Software configurations and versions can differ between practices. (N.B. The data inclusions would now need to be updated to comply with the latest NSF requirements but the principles are the same.)

An approach outlined for the Fylde programme is structured as follows by:

- *setting up the EMIS audit according to the policy definitions.* Noting the audit requirements of the policy (the outputs) and confirming the required inputs are there to meet them, i.e. coding consistency (ensuring the Read Codes used to record the data are the same as those used in any searches and audits and that all the necessary codes are included)
- *designing a template to assist in the capture of the data.* Matching the codes used in the template to those being used by the EMIS audit. The specified codes can be incorporated into existing templates or new templates can be designed.

The codes are specified in the policy produced by the PCG (see previous chapters).

In addition during the year of the CHD programme it is possible to monitor data quality and also to target activity by:

- *setting up searches to detect and then correct likely coding inconsistencies.* These may be peculiar to each practice and searches should be designed accordingly. Codes designated within the policy are used in preference. For example, a history and symptom code for 'history of hypertension 14A2' may have been used instead of 'essential hypertension G20' a disease code. Searching on the former code and replacing with the latter
- *adding overdue diary markers for priority patients and those with incomplete data recorded* – for example, patients with CHD not recorded as taking aspirin.

This would help to highlight patients when they attend and allows staff to either correct the data or issue a prescription. This helps to direct clinical activity during the programme and identify priority groups from the audits. Such markers appear as 'flashing reminders' on the patient record.

Other examples for marking would be patients:

- with uncontrolled hypertension
- with diabetes
- smoking but not received advice or offered cessation support
- with lipid levels outside the target ranges.

Prioritising and targeting such groups will depend on local circumstances and the prevalence of disease. Ensuring removal of these markers once an intervention is made is part of maintaining the system and can be done either at the time of seeing a patient or by searches later on.

Use of an associated 'recall schedule' on the system can be used to automatically cancel the diary markers once a code for an intervention is added. N.B. Using too many of these markers reduces their impact and they may get ignored.

When adding a code to the patient record if there is a 'recall schedule' set for that code, the diary date for that code will be cancelled. Further actions can also be set, e.g. adding a further diary entry for the future.

Adding a recall schedule can be done from the main menu:

DT: Dictionaries and Templates
B: Recall Schedules
A: Add a Schedule

Viewing and editing of the recall schedule can be done through this menu.

Setting up the CHD 'audit' in EMIS

Note, the term 'audit(s)' also has a meaning specific to the EMIS system and is used to describe that part of the searching facility that looks at groups of patients rather than individuals (then called 'searches'). The term appears in menus on the system in this context.

This audit feature allows the building of a series of interlinked searches and criteria looking at whole populations. Both the construction of the audit and the methods of displaying the results will allow powerful analysis of such groups.

A number of steps are followed:

- *creating a 'Target Population' for the audit*. This limits the focus of the searches to a specified group – in this case patients with CHD up to the age of 75 (this does not mean older patients are excluded from treatment)
- *creating the audit*. This involves adding the codes specified in the PCG table to the audit criteria
- *running the audit*. More complex audits can take some time to run and can possibly slow the system during a busy day. They can be set to run automatically each night so giving an up-to-date assessment each morning
- *producing the audit results*. The results can be output in a variety of ways, exported to other software, e.g. Excel spreadsheet, or included in a structured 'report' generated from the EMIS word processor.

Creating a 'Target Population' for the audit

This is the first step and is simply performing a search and storing the result for use by the audit. All further actions of the audit will look at this defined group. This needs to be done prior to building the audit and thought should be given to the features to be included in this initial search. In this case it is all patients in the practice ever coded as having IHD.

From the main menu follow: ST, C

Practice Audit	
A Manage Target Populations	
B Audits and Reports	

Option A selects the 'target population manager'.

Audit Target Populations
A Build a target population
R Results of target population search
V View Target population parameters
D Delete Target population
E Edit Target population parameters
M Build a target population using modified parameters

Building the population uses the usual 'Search and Statistics' menus. The target population includes all patients in the practice with IHD, i.e. coded as G3 (Read Version 5).

A Add Feature	**C** Cancel Feature	**I** Insert Feature	**R** Code Review
O Alter Operator	**X** View Exclusions	**D** Alter a Date Range	

Feature	Date Range	Operator
A Currently registered (regular -pd)		SHARED

Adding the feature brings up the next menu. This offers a comprehensive set of options for features that can be included within a search – the Read Codes being selected by highlighting the section marked CC (Classification Codes) and pressing Enter.

This brings up the familiar Read Code browser.

```
          Select Entry : ▮

Enter free text, line label, or move cursor

A Allergy                          B O/E - blood pressure reading
C Common entries                   E Clinical Summary Coding
F Forms & Insurance                G Full Classification
H Family history                   I Immunisation
L Patients Problem List            M Child Health Care
N Cervical smear taken             O Oral contraceptive
P Preventive Care                  Q Clinical Protocols
R Referral For Further Care        S Surgical Procedures
T Templates                        V Values & Investigations
W Warfarin monitoring        <T> X Cause of Death
Y Letter Sent to Patient
```

The code can be selected by entering text or the code itself at the 'Select Entry' prompt. In this case IHD or G3 will select the code. If the code selected is a higher-level code you will be offered the option to exclude certain codes – codes included are marked with a 'Y' by default. The codes can be included or excluded by following the screen prompts. In this case all lower level codes are required and they are included simply by pressing Enter. The option to limit the search to a date range is presented – this can limit the search to a given period. Look for only the most recent entry – in this case no date range is requested as all patients who have ever had IHD are being included.

A further option is then offered to restrict the search to 'active problems' as marked in the EMIS record. This defaults to 'No' as required in this audit where all records of IHD are to be included.

The next option sets the 'Operator' for the search – in this case the code is 'SHARED'.

```
You have selected the feature :

   Ischaemic heart disease

You must now select the 'Operator' for this feature

Select one of the following : ▮

 A  SHARED. This indicates that the group of patients you are searching
    for must all share this feature. Any patient who does not have this
    feature will not be included in the final group.

 B  EXCLUDED . Any patient who has this feature will be excluded from
    the final group.

 C  EITHER/OR. You may wish to find a group of patients with a number of
    alternative features. Patients will be included in the final group
    if they have any of these features. If they have NONE of the features
    with this operator they will not appear in the final group.
```

This then returns to the original 'search parameter' page when further features can be added if necessary. If no more are to be added, following the screen prompts then allows the search to be completed and saved. You are required to provide a title and this should reflect the content and purpose of the audit to help identify it to others.

In this case 'PCG CHD audit population' is entered. This is then saved into the relevant directory for further access. The section marked EMIS audit target populations is password protected on some systems and may prevent easy access to the searches if stored there.

In saving the search the option to 'run now' can be taken. The system then returns back to the 'Target Populations' menu.

Using the F1 key to return to the 'Practice Audit' menu the second menu choice, 'Audits and Reports', can now be selected.

```
Audit Management                                              [⊡⊡]

A  Add an Audit·                      P  Perform an Audit
R  Audit Results                      D  Delete an Audit
E  Edit Audit                         V  View Parameters
S  Slide Dates                        N  Run Audit Nightly
B  Build/Edit audit reports

Title                                                    Nightly ?
```

The Audit Management menu

Option A (to add an audit) is selected. There will be a reminder to build the target population, as described above.

The previous search is then selected from where it was stored – the pages offered will now be familiar. The menu then offers the addition of audit features. This allows for complex combinations of parameters to be selected.

```
Building Or Editing Groups Of Features To Audit              [⊡⊡]
Target Population : PCG CHD Audit population

A  Add a Feature to Audit            D  Delete a Feature from Audit
O  Add 'OR' operators                S  Add 'Shared' or 'AND' operators
E  Alter Date range                  N  Add 'NOT' operators
B  Edit an abbreviated description    T  Tabular default display
X  View Exclusions

   Feature                                        Abbreviation

1  Coronary artery operations                     Coronary Art Ops
```

The features of the audit are now 'built' in an iterative process. This can be a some-what laborious process for a complex audit and it is worth setting aside sufficient time if the process is not familiar. With repetition comes speed. For the novice it can be worth setting up 'mock audits' to get the feel of the software before finalising the content. These test audits can be easily deleted.

The steps are generally straightforward. There are often search 'pitfalls' that become apparent. In the case of this audit it can be seen with the selection of drugs that appear in more than one BNF chapter.

As an example of adding an audit feature the code for 'coronary artery operations 792' will be added.

Choose Option A to add a feature; this produces the feature selection list. As before the Read Codes are under section CC (Classification Codes). Selecting this and entering '792' at the 'Select Entry' prompt brings up the Read Code list. On selecting the top-level code 792 the option of including/excluding codes and adding a date range are offered. Having selected the required ranges the next page prompts for an abbreviation (up to 18 characters) for the audit feature that will appear in the 'tabular display'. These abbreviations could be planned in advance so as the meaning is clear to a variety of users.

```
 Building Or Editing Groups Of Features To Audit
Target Population : PCG CHD Audit population

A  Add a Feature to Audit            D  Delete a Feature from Audit
O  Add 'OR' operators                S  Add 'Shared' or 'AND' operators
E  Alter Date range                  N  Add 'NOT' operators
B  Edit an abbreviated description   T  Tabular default display
X  View Exclusions

   Feature                                         Abbreviation

1  Coronary artery operations                      Coronary Art Ops
```

If errors are made it is possible to delete a feature using Option D.

Adding features with numerical values also prompts for the upper and lower ranges to be included.

Further features are added until all are complete. Pressing Enter/Return completes the building process. You are then offered the options for eventual display of the results. It is often simplest to accept the default values suggested in brackets.

Depending on the audit output you are then able to select either 'patient numbers' of the number of instances of audit features (i.e. the incidence).

The audit is then given a title. Again this should clearly state the nature of the audit for other users of the system. Following this is the option to set all dates in the audit relative to a specific date – pressing Enter will set today's date.

It is possible to return and edit the features of the audit if mistakes become apparent.

The completed audit will then appear in the audit management listing.

There is an option to run the audits each night and the system tags the audit list for audits set to run in this way.

The option to 'slide dates' is used to update the original dates set. The 'sliding' updates both the target population and audit features and can be important to include new patients in the target population who were not identified on the system when the original population was built.

The complete audit listing can be viewed in a series of pages to check that all parameters are included.

```
13 Patients taking Oral Anticoagulants  Between 1.8.2000 and 2.10.2000
14 Adverse reaction to aspirin
15 Serum cholesterol
16 Serum LDL cholesterol level 3.1-10
17 Serum LDL cholesterol level 1-3 (most recent -Serum LDL cholesterol level)
18 Patients taking Drugs Used In Hyperlipidaemia (-exclusions)
   Between 1.8.2000 and 2.10.2000
19 Systolic blood pressure
20 Diastolic blood pressure
21 Patients with either 19 20
22 Systolic blood pressure 141-300
23 Diastolic blood pressure 86-250
```

Having spent all the time constructing the audit the output can receive some attention.

There is a neat and little-used feature in the audit management menu:

Option B – Build/edit audit reports
This uses the EMIS word processor to create a document that can be printed out to include added commentary and observations.

The data from the audit is 'merged' into the document. These results can be placed within sentences to create an updateable report document that can be far more readable than a set of tables and statistics. Some familiarity in using the EMIS word processor is helpful. The Shift+F5 function is most important in selecting data results from the audit to be merged in to the document.

A number of report documents can be created for an audit and this allows quite sophisticated selection of incidence and prevalence. The full details of how to use the report manager can be found in the EMIS manuals or as often by trial and error.

The audit must be run again before the reports can be printed or if any audit features have been changed.

The Audit report output is selected as follows:

1   From the Audit Management menu:
        Page down to show the audit title required.
        R – Audit Results.
        Enter a letter to select the audit required and press Enter.

2   The next menu offers a selection of result outputs, choose option:
    R – Audit reports
    The reports built for the audit are shown as a numbered list with their titles.
3   Select the number of the report to be printed and press Return.

This displays the usual menu used to output from EMIS. Choose the printer or other methods of output from the list in the usual way.

A simpler and more familiar way to view the results is via Option R in the Audit Management menu.

Selecting 'tabular printout of audit' allows the table to be printed or displayed. The option 'export to ASCII file' allows the data to be transferred to a file that can be used in other software such as Excel spreadsheet. This is a simple process – some technical 'path names' are required depending on the set up of the practice system, but these are usually straightforward. The option to export to Excel offers far more powerful analysis and presentation methods and can be used to advantage by the PCG to compare and feedback practice data.

A template to complement the audit requirements

Most practices will be familiar with the use of templates on the EMIS system (see below). The process of creating them will not be extensively covered here.

Existing templates are likely to be in use covering areas such as hypertension, heart failure and CHD. Existing templates would need to be checked to see that they include the correct codes specified.

Template Entry			
Prompt	Result	Date	Last Recorded Entry
IHD diagnosis			Acute Mi 14.9.2000
Angina pectoris			Angina 2.9.2000
Coronary Art Ops			Coronary Art Ops -----
Cerebrovasc dis,			Cerebrovasc dis, -----
Artery/Vessl dis			Saddle embolus 30.9.1999
Atrial fib+flutt			Atrial fib+flutt -----
Heart failure			Heart failure -----
Smoking Status			Never 25.9.2000
Smoking Advice			Health ed. – sm 25.9.2000

```
A Acute Mi           F Subsequent MI        K I H D Nos
B Ihd Other          G Comp Post Mi
C Old Mi             H Cardiac syndrome X
D Angina pectoris    I Postoperative MI
E Chronic Ihd        J I H D
```

Some practices choose to provide a set of smaller templates for use within a disease area, for example a larger template can be used at an initial assessment including data that is not likely to need regular changes and an additional template used during a follow-up contact that includes the codes that will vary e.g. blood pressure, urinalysis, symptoms, lab results etc. The codes included in each will need to be the same and data entered in one template is then automatically included when using any other template containing that code. These smaller templates can be easier to complete during a consultation.

It is also important to maintain the template listings and to modify or delete older or unused templates that may contain redundant coding. Templates used for other disease areas may also contain redundant codes – this can be another cause of deteriorating data quality. Any member of staff providing templates needs to be aware of these issues.

The template building/editing area is usually found from the main menu under:

    DT: Dictionaries and Templates
    C: Codes, Templates and Protocols
    E: Edit access screen/Forms/Templates
    T: Templates

Experienced practices may have configured their own structure for the template selection menu rather than using the default version supplied with the system. In this case a separate section may already be available for 'cardiovascular disease' or similar.

It is worth remembering that the title for a template can appear in more than one section of template selection pages as it is simply a pointer to the template. The template itself is stored elsewhere.

By using this combination of template to input data for the audit, the audit itself to monitor change over time and diary reminders to highlight priorities for attention, the CHD prevention activity within the practice can be improved. Feeding back progress to the clinical team is obviously important.

There are a number of other ways of configuring the EMIS system and though more complicated to set up they can be more powerful. The use of 'protocols' on the system can automatically check for missing codes within records and prompt accordingly. These can be set to run each time a prescription is issued. The process is appropriate for those more experienced in the use of the system and comfortable in building the 'protocols' themselves.

Offering full care for CHD will often include other factors beyond those included in a given audit or template and new clinical users may need to be reminded of this.

The new requirements of the NSF for CHD (2000) are now a priority. Reference to work on this and considerations for practices are included later, including template content for use across a PCG and codes that have been selected by some groups elsewhere. The coding matrix includes a wide selection of Read Codes that can be included in templates and audits. *See* also Appendix C.

Part Three

Where do we go from here?

Chapter 9

Future PCG developments for coding CHD

The National Service Framework for Coronary Heart Disease (NSF CHD)

In common with many PCGs and medical audit advisory groups (MAAGs), Fylde chose to implement a programme concentrating on CHD early on in the development of a health improvement programme (HImP). Data input, collection and computer analysis has been in progress for a number of years. Decisions on coding and audit criteria have been taken at a local level.

The NHS NSF CHD developments have since added specified requirements; targets and milestones for CHD management in both primary and secondary care now include a specified annual audit requirement.

As with the Fylde programme parts of this new audit requirement are being met within existing activity but there are areas that are not included, e.g. heart failure and primary prevention.

It will be important for PCGs to identify these gaps and modify their data collection and analysis accordingly.

As most practices will not be starting afresh on their clinical coding of CHD and may not have been consistent in their use of codes so far there will be a need for tidying and 'cleaning' the data. To assist in this process, guidance and agreement on minimum data sets is needed and early attention to this can prevent extra work later on. In trying to address the problem coding formularies are proliferating across the country. If not decided at national level then PCGs are well placed to provide the lead and can draw on previous work done by CHDGP and the newly formed PRIMIS project based at Nottingham University.

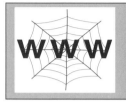

WWW link

On the Web pages linked to this book you will find links to the PRIMIS web site at www.primis.nhs.uk/

This web site provides a download (pdf) of a data query set as used for MIQUEST based on data collection projects and a summary of the Read Code specification to support the NSF CHD.

Involvement in the full PRIMIS project requires the appointment and funding of a facilitator at local level. With improvement in data quality and information many PCGs have found this investment worthwhile.

The NHS information authority (NHSIA) are likely to give further guidance on data collection and coding to support this and forthcoming NSFs.

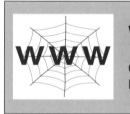

WWW link

On the Web pages linked to this book you will find links to the NHS Information Authority web site at http://www.nhsia.nhs.uk

However most practices and PCGs are keen to progress and will already have made their own coding decisions.

Where local codes have been developed or 'own-codes' created on a practice computer system, attention will need to be given to standardisation across a PCG area.

Clinical coding and clinical governance

Codes used in one practice will have their own context and significance and may represent completely different clinical activity between practices.

In one practice a code for 'Health education – smoking' might represent a brief sentence of simple advice to stop smoking, while in another practice it may only be used to represent inclusion in a comprehensive smoking cessation programme.

For the purposes of clinical governance this will present a problem and a challenge as the presence of a code cannot be assumed to represent a particular clinical activity.

Validating such data and its link to real clinical activity is an issue for the future.

This aspect of coding also raises concerns around medico–legal validity and recording of care in an electronic form – it is important not to think that coding in the record is the same as providing a complete and accurate record of a consultation.

As mentioned before, clinicians and managers should not assume that a local audit or audit features includes all the important requirements of full care in a particular disease area.

This is exemplified by the national audit for NSF CHD – for audit purposes the population analysis is limited to those aged 35–74.

Patients outside this age range should not be denied similar screening and treatments but there is an obvious risk that they may become a lower priority group.

Fulfilling an audit requirement may indicate the provision of adequate care but it is not the same and unless the audit was specifically designed to include all the elements of good care this limitation needs to be remembered.

To assist clinical governance there may be a temptation to proliferate all manner of codes to represent the minutiae of clinical activity. At present most doctors will document this in the form of a narrative or free text entry in the computer record. Hopefully there are few PCGs who will want their clinicians distracted from real patient care by the need to enter codes for all such activity. A realistic compromise will be needed.

Where possible a good principle to follow is that data should be collected as a by-product of the provision and recording of good clinical care and not by having coding as a separate activity.

Some agreement on these issues will be required but is seldom included in any data collection programme relating to the activity of primary care clinicians. For this reason audits are sometimes restricted to areas related to discrete activity, the presence of a prescription for a drug or a blood pressure reading. These are examples of data generated as a by-product, i.e. simply by issuing a prescription or recording BP on the patient record in a consultation. No extra work has been required other than would have taken place anyway.

Moving from a local policy to the NSF CHD

There has been a wealth of evidence-based information available for CHD prevention highlighting the shortcomings in the management of risk factors.

The local policy in Fylde as in many PCGs aimed to focus on the secondary prevention of CHD (i.e. preventing the progression of disease in those already symptomatic).

Secondary prevention is confirmed as the priority in the NSF particularly in groups at highest risk, e.g. diabetic and hypertensive patients.

The NSF approaches the problem by requiring the provision of a 'disease register'. This concept appears to be dating in an age when most GPs are essentially managing large databases relating to their patients.

The issues now are more to do with the 'quality of data' contained within this database rather than just compiling a simplistic 'register'. Nonetheless a complete database of the relevant patients is the important requirement, and 'register' is the term likely to be used synonymously with 'database'.

Beyond any local scheme for secondary prevention the NSF will also require the identification of patients at risk from CHD but not yet developing symptoms – 'primary prevention'. Calculation of such an individual's absolute 10-year risk of developing CHD is recommended. From the NSF a suggested tool to assist in this is the Framingham risk score.

Such a calculation tool is available as a paper chart as the Joint British Societies Coronary Risk Prediction Chart now included with the BNF (British National Formulary).

Practice computer systems now include calculation tools. The EMIS system contains the required facility within the software and by constructing a template this score can be quickly calculated. A graphical version is also available in the Windows version of *Mentor* on the EMIS system.

Free PC programmes are also available for this purpose (*see* Appendix B).

Building a true PCG-wide CHD 'register'

It will not be long before the PCGs will be required to collate the data for their district relating to CHD indicators for the purposes of the annual audit. The PCG will expect complete, reliable and accurate information and will rely upon practices to provide it. Is this data going to be reliable?

Most practices will need to give an honest answer to the following questions.

'Is it certain that all patients who have ever suffered from CHD are accurately coded as such on the practice computer system?'

'Is there an effective system in place that will capture the data for all future patients developing CHD?'

If the honest answer to both of these questions is *'yes'* then such practices are in an enviable minority, for most will have a patchy database not developed systematically and with insufficient recording and accuracy of historical data.

There may or may not be systematic recording of data for new patients diagnosed with CHD.

All is not lost however and by using some simple techniques and creative use of existing data a majority of CHD patients can be identified and coded as such.

Historical data is likely to be a problem. In the evolution to 'paper-light' practices it is hoped that all the data from the Lloyd-George records has been captured effectively. How complete and reliable this process has been is not fully known and consequently errors in such coding are possible.

Errors have arisen because of poor quality of the paper record, poor training of the person interpreting and transferring the information and little standardisation of clinical codes used in the process.

If it is felt within a practice or PCG that electronic data is not trustworthy the time-consuming and expensive prospect of re-examining notes has to be faced – but this should be a last resort. Summarisation of paper records requires the application of appropriate standards

Create a CHD register by using your prescribing data

A recent study published in the *BMJ* (Sept 2000, **321**: 548–50) looked at this problem.

Although it may not be possible to assume all the conclusions are applicable across the country, the results are encouraging even for a practice not using a computer to prescribe.

Most practices now record both their acute and repeat prescriptions on computer and this data is widely believed to be of relatively high quality. Searching for the G3 code or nitrate (as suggested in the NSF) does miss almost 30% of patients with IHD but much higher percentages can be detected by adding further drugs to the search.

From the Battersea Research Group figures, adding four additional drugs to the search for G3 or nitrate, aspirin, Digoxin, Atenolol and statins will identify about 90% of IHD patients.

Search Structure	Sensitivity % (95% CI) (n=93)
With G3 Read Code	47 (36-59)
G3 or nitrate	73 (59-87)
G3 or nitrate or aspirin	89 (83-96)
G3 or nitrate or aspirin or atenolol	94 (87-100)
G3 or nitrate or aspirin or atenolol or digoxin or statin	96 (89-100)

The encouraging fact is that non-computerised practices could therefore identify (albeit more slowly) a similar high proportion of their IHD patients using just their repeat prescribing data.

Recent work has suggested that the vast majority of these patients attend during the year and the further 10% can hopefully be detected and identified using an opportunistic approach over time.

Primary prevention: the Framingham risk score

Although this area is not the immediate priority in implementing the NSF or a local PCG policy the use of a computer calculation tool has proved appealing to both clinicians and patients, though caution has to be exercised in its use to avoid creating undue anxiety in essentially healthy patients.

Freestanding computer calculation tools are available free of charge. Practice computers also include this feature including the EMIS software which integrates well into the clinical system.

It is relatively easy to set up and use and has been helpful in increasing awareness of the CHD programme for clinicians.

The ability to identify and modify risk factors can be helpful in motivating patients. Additional risk factors may need to be considered such as poor family history of CHD and very high BMI (over 35). The original Framingham study looked at the 30–74 year age group.

Patients with a 10-year risk of 30% or greater are identified as the priority – it will be possible for a PCG to show improvements in risk over time as a result of interventions, drug treatments, e.g. statins, and other risk factor modifications.

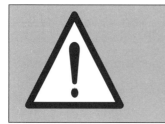

Remember this calculation should not be used in those already suffering from IHD or other cardiovascular disease – this group would be included under secondary prevention strategies.

Implementing the Framingham score on an EMIS system

This is an example of using this score by integrating Read Codes already on the patient record. The EMIS system method is straightforward and requires the building of a template on the system.

EMIS has created its own code for the 10-year absolute risk of CHD and has included codes on the system to aid in the calculation.

The codes EMISFR3, EMISFR4, represent 10-year and estimated 10-year risks. As can be seen these are not special codes, but do not have the typical Read Code structure.

The template should be created to include the following codes as a minimum. These codes can also be included as prompts in an existing template and will still allow the calculation.

Template Prompt	Read Code (Version 5)
Smoking status	(Egton320 (Code may have been converted
Diabetes	(C10)
Left Ventricle Hypertrophy on ECG	(324)
Serum Cholesterol	(44P)
HDL cholesterol	(44P5)
Cholesterol/ration	(EMISTCH)
Systolic Blood pressure	(2469)
Diastolic Blood Pressure	(246A) (Not used in the calculation)
10-year risk (estimate)	EMISFR4
10-year risk	EMISFR3

If electronically linked to the pathology laboratory, cholesterol results will automatically be included if they are filed and coded appropriately on the system – codes used by local laboratories may differ.

On the EMIS system templates are stored in the usual section, from the main menu page, under DT, C, E, T.

The main steps are:

1   Select the template title (Framingham risk score) and insert in the access screen where you prefer.
2   Edit the template using the Edit menu choosing options to prompt for a date.
3   Add the prompts in the template using the codes above.
4   Save the template.
5   Test the template using a 'dummy' patient.

When using the calculation a box will appear with codes for EMISFR3, 4. It will show whether any assumed values have been used in the calculation before you accept the score.

To calculate the actual risk would require a cholesterol/HDL result but the system can estimate this if the result is not available.

For full details on setting up a template refer to your EMIS manual or local trainer.

What data to record for NSF CHD

Without being too philosophical and not intending to state the obvious, but in order to give an answer a question is needed.

So often however questions are not specified prior to collecting data. Data collection proceeds but when it comes to drawing on the data it becomes obvious that data was being collected for non-existent questions or data being collected is not capable of providing useful answers to important questions.

This issue is important in healthcare as data is often captured during the limited time spent in consultation with a patient.

The NSF places an emphasis on audit, the audit requirements are set at different levels for practice and PCG but both will be drawing on the data set held at practice level.

These audit specifications can be used to provide the 'questions' and so help to determine the specific data to capture and therefore dictate the content of templates, searches and EMIS audits.

The CHD secondary prevention audit specifies:
(NSF Annual Clinical Audit – secondary prevention)

1 Record the number and proportion of the registered population aged 35–74 years with:
    a) recognised coronary heart disease
    b) transient ischaemic attack (TIA)/ischaemic stroke
    c) peripheral vascular disease.
2 For each of these groups (1 a–c), record the number and proportion of people whose records document:
    a) advice about use of aspirin
    b) serum cholesterol below 5 mmol/l
    c) smoking status and, for smokers, delivery of, or referral for, appropriate advice
    d) blood pressure less than 150 mmHg systolic and 90 mmHg diastolic.
3 Number and proportion of people aged 35–74 years with a history of acute Ml in the past 12 months, prescribed beta-blockers.
4 Number and proportion of people with confirmed left ventricular systolic dysfunction prescribed an ACE inhibitor.
5 Number and proportion of people over 60-years old with atrial fibrillation prescribed warfarin or aspirin (or with documented advice to take aspirin regularly).

As a minimum, codes will be required for each feature listed which can then be incorporated into an EMIS audit as outlined previously.

Local decisions may be taken on whether to provide a ready-made template and audit for practices to use on their EMIS system. It does seem a duplication of work if it is left to individual practices to complete.

As with the Fylde PCG programme a suggested table of codes is an option. Some PCGs are choosing to specify and disseminate a data entry template. The option for practices remains to use their own templates as long as the coding is consistent with the PCG requirements.

Increasing use of MIQUEST software can save work at practice level and speed data delivery to the PCG.

Agreeing codes for the PCG implementation of the NSF

National standardisation is the real requirement for clinical coding of the NSF CHD and future NSFs. Until this is confirmed local decisions will be required to provide coding consistency across a PCG or health authority. Local implementation teams for the NSF should be involved in this process (*see* Chapter 5).

An input template is the preferred method on many systems to draw codes together and present them to the clinician when gathering data during a consultation. Agreeing the content of such a template is not always straightforward.

Reaching agreement on the use and 'meaning' of codes is not always as simple as initially thought and debates about coding semantics can become involved. The grey areas of investigation and diagnosis are familiar to all clinicians. It can be difficult to choose codes that accurately represent these realities.

These limitations accepted, a systematic analysis of the requirements of the NSF CHD for audit and clinical implementation can be made. These can then be mapped against the current codes available or which have been used elsewhere.

Blackpool PCG has done work on a coding table to assist in this process across clinical systems. This is shown in full at the end of this section.

- The main audit criteria are identified and listed in the table.
- Coding lists are collected from various sources.
- Codes are matched within the table.

Evaluation of coding importance is carried out (group agreement).

This method allows coding trends and anomalies to be identified. There may be obvious coding gaps where criteria are listed but no codes are matched to them. The matrix opposite continues to be refined until all the factors of the NSF are included to the satisfaction of the local implementation teams.

After a thorough search, if no suitable Read Code is found it may mean a code does not exist. Agreement will then be needed on a suitable 'in-house' code to be used. This process can be used for future NSFs.

Having determined the coding content and structure, work can begin on building the templates to assist with capture of the relevant data.

Whether employing a PCG-based data extraction method or using tools such as MIQUEST, a systematic approach is required to ensure the production of valid information.

The following table captures many of the available Read Codes presently in use in the area of coronary heart disease management. *See* also Appendix C for some agreed data inclusions for CHD.

NSF CHD Codings

Patients 35–74 (for audit purposes)

BP <150/90, target 140/85

ly=last year

B=Basic

I=Intermediate

A=Advanced

Data Criteria	Leeds	Fylde 5-Byte	PRIMIS	Web search 4-Byte	Web search 5-Byte	NSF CHD 4-Byte	NSF CHD 5-Byte	Audit	Essential	Desirable	Not needed
Patient Details											
Age DOB			B								
Sex			B								
Modifiable Risk Factors											
Body Mass Index	22K		B (ly)	22K (plus value)				Y			
Systolic blood pressure	2469	2469			2469						
Diastolic blood pressure	246A	246A			246A						
Smoking status			B (ly)	137+ (plus value)				Y			
Current smoker	137R	137R	B					Y			
Current non-smoker	137L	137L	B								
Health Education – smoking	6791										
Referral to cessation service								Y (ly)			
NRT / Zyban											
Dietary advice given	6799			8CA4							
Pt advised re reducing diet				none	8CA40						
Pt adv re low cholesterol diet				none	8CA47						
Pt advised re low salt diet				none	8CA48						
Alcohol Intake	Egton418										
Health Education – alcohol	6792										
Health Education – exercise	6798										
Exercise advice given				8CA5							
Current level of physical activity	138				138			Y			

NSF CHD Codings

Patients 35–74 (for audit purposes) ly=last year

BP <150/90, target 140/85 B=Basic I=Intermediate A=Advanced

Data Criteria	Leeds	Fylde 5-Byte	PRIMIS	Web search 4-Byte	Web search 5-Byte	CHD NSF 4-Byte	CHD NSF 5-Byte	Audit	Essential	Desirable	Not Needed
Unmodifiable Risk Factors											
Patient with CHD	G3 12C	G3	B	G4+	G3+	G4	G3	Y			
Family history of CHD < 60			I	12C2	12C2						
Family history of CVA/stroke				12C4	12C4						
Had MI		G30 G31 G32				G41	G31				
MI < 60			I	14A3	14A3						
MI > 60				14A4	14A4						
MI in last year			B	14AH	14AH			Y			
LV Dysfunction								Y			
Angina			I			G44	G33				
History of angina				14A5	14A5						
History of angina in last yr			B	14AJ	14AJ						
BP recorded		2469/246A B (ly)									
Ever/latest systolic BP		2469/246A									
>140 or diastolic > 85			B								
Hypertension			B								
BP			A	246+ (plus value)							
Atrial fibrillation		G573	A			G67	G573	Y			
Cerebrovascular disease				G71+	G6+			Y			
TIA			A	G74	G65+						
History of TIA			14AB	14AB				Y			

Stroke/CVA			A	G75	G66+	G75	G66	Y
History of stroke				14A7	14A7			
History of stroke in last yr				14AK	14AK			
Atherosclerosis/PVD			A			G81	G70	Y
PVD NOS ?no other symptoms				G86	G73z			
PVD NOS ?no other symptoms				G86z	G73zz			
Intermittent claudication				G85	G73z1			
Spasm of peripheral artery				none	G73z2			
Thromboangiitis obliterans				G861	G731			
Heart failure			A	G6A+	G58+	G6A	G58	Y
Diabetes Mellitus			B	C2	C10			Y
Annual diabetic review								
Blood glucose result								Y
Treatment/monitoring								
Aspirin prophylaxis	8B63		B	8B63				Y
Aspirin adverse effect	TJ53	TJ53–1						
Aspirin refused	8I38							
Aspirin contraindicated	8I24							
Over counter aspirin	8B3T							
Patient advised re OTC med				8CA3				
Anticoagulant prophylaxis				8B61				
Warfarin if AF			A					Y
Beta blocker prophylaxis	8B69							
Beta blocker contra-indicated	8I26							
Beta blocker refused	8I36							
Beta blocker not indicated	8I62							
Adverse reaction to beta blocker	TJC6							
Total cholesterol	44P	44P	B (ly)	44P+ (plus value)				Y
HDL				44P5				
LDL				44P6	44P3			
LDL <3.1 recorded	44P6							
Triglycerides				44Q				
Cholesterol target			A					Y

NSF CHD Codings

ly=last year

Patients 35–74 (for audit purposes)   B=Basic

BP <150/90, target 140/85   I=Intermediate

A=Advanced

Data Criteria	Leeds	Fylde 5-Byte	PRIMIS	Web search 4-Byte 773+	Web search 5-Byte 792+	CHD NSF	Essential	Desirable	Not Needed
Coronary artery surgery		792							
had angioplasty									
had angiogram									
CABG									
valve replacement									
Cardiology out-pt appt									
Standard ECG	3212								
Exercise ECG	3213					Y			
Echo	5853								
Stress test									
Angiogram						Y			
Drug therapy list									
Beta blocker			I						
ACEI			I			Y			
Statin			B			Y			
Urine protein	467+								
Urine glucose	466+								
Cardiac rehab						Y			
Written self-care plan						Y			
Advised re local support groups									
CPR training for family									
CHD risk assessment						Y			
CHD Monitoring	662N								
Occupations	O								

Chapter 10

Conclusions

This book has taken you from the theoretical potential of computer-based electronic disease registers to the brink of the reality. Along the way we have recognised the many problems and barriers and sought to identify tools, methods and solutions to address them.

We have taken you through a multistage process:

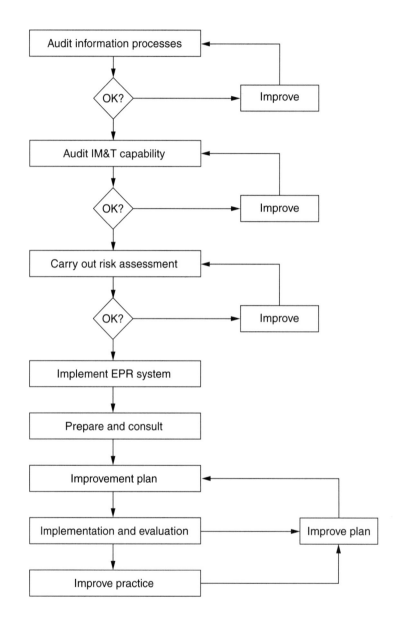

However, this is an over-simplistic representation of the process as we have tried to show.

For further resources to help you address these issues, please refer to the appendices and to the book's web site which may be found at: www.radcliffe-oxford.com/edr or www.alangillies.co.uk/echd/.

Appendices:

Further resources

Appendix A
VISION guidance for the NSF

VISION

NSF for CHD

Health Informatics Programme

National Service Framework for Coronary Heart Disease

User Guide

KMAN111

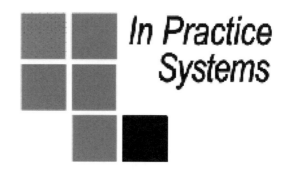
*In Practice
Systems*

Date		Contents	Authors
Nov 2000	1	V.HIP NSF CHD Guideline	Emma Brezan
			Alison Young
14.11.00	2	-ditto-	Ed. J Thomas

Table of editions.

Contents

HIP NSF for CHD   135
    Introduction   135

Clinical Audit   135
    NSF Clinical Audits   135
    To import the NSF Clinical Audits   137
    Make CHD reminders active   138
    Generation of the NSF audits   139

Problem orientated approach to chronic disease registers   140
    Why create a problem?   140
    To create a problem for patients with evidence or risk of
        CHD   140

Guidelines   143
    Import the CHD Guideline and Report   143
    What the CHD Guideline contains   144
    Add Read Code triggers   145
    What happens once the Guidelines have triggers 146

HIP NSF for CHD

Introduction

The National Service Framework (NSF) for Coronary Heart Disease (CHD) sets national standards to establish performance measures against which progress will be measured and monitored.

Patients' details, treatment or care provided and health outcomes must be recorded consistently and comprehensively to support direct patient care, so the information can be queried or analysed to monitor performance against specific targets.

HIP for CHD is a comprehensive Health Informatics Programme to support the information requirements of the NSF in primary care. It is a practical example of clinical governance.

In Practice Systems Ltd have provided a number of tools to enable practices to capture and analyse the data required by the NSF.

- **Clinical Audit** – will find patients with data for coronary heart disease, arterial disease and high risk factors, and will enable the attachment of yellow reminders.
- **Problem orientated approach to Chronic Disease Registers** – will attach a problem called NSFCHD to each patient. This will trigger the NSFCHD Guideline when that patient is selected.
- **Guidelines** – This is a data entry guideline to encourage the recording of good quality information for the mangement of those patients with or at risk of CHD.
- **EMIS** – 'Protocol' released July 2001.

Clinical Audit

NSF Clinical Audits

A new audit NSF for CHD has been developed and can be downloaded from www.inps.co.uk, or from the monthly CD which contains your Drug Dictionary and other files, and imported into the Clinical Audit module.

This audit should be generated each month to provide the information required by the NSF for CHD.

The purpose of the Clinical Audit module is to provide monthly statistics of data, collected from the pre-defined searches. This can stretch back several years to provide a snapshot in time and enable trends to be detected.

The Clinical Audit can be run at any time during the month, when it will collect up the statistics for the previous month, for example, running it on 3 October will collect statistics up until 30 September.

Groups of patients are created, matching the various criteria within each area, for example, 'Patients with Existing CHD', and various sub-divisions, such as 'Patients with Existing CHD who have had an ECG'.

The search list can be expanded to reveal levels of information, the lower levels represented by an indent, so in the following example, Cardiovascular Disease is the parent line for Existing CHD:

Source – National Service Framework (in blue)
Clinical area – Coronary Heart Disease (in red)
Clinical category (in green) – CHD Existing – Monitoring
Searches (in grey) – Patients with Existing CHD
Sub-levels of searches (in grey)
Patients who have had an ECG
Patients with a normal ECG on ACE inhibitors

Clicking will expand or collapse a line. At the lowest level, a double click displays the patients within that group.

The count of patients is expressed as a percentage of a base population. In most cases this is the whole practice population, but in others it may only be those, for example, diagnosed with hypertension, or all female patients. The base population on which an audit group's percentages are based (by default) can easily be found by looking at the base population figure on its parent line.

The results of each audit group can be viewed graphically by age/sex, prevalence (over time) and incidence (changes over time). You may choose bar graphs or line charts, and determine the colours with which graphs are illustrated. The figures can be varied, for instance by patient count, or percentage of base population, and the base population can also be varied.

Search results can be exported to third-party packages such as Excel.

For more details about Clinical Audit, visit the on-screen help.

To import the NSF Clinical Audits

1 Put Clinical Audit in Maintenance mode, either by clicking on 📇 or select File – Maintenance Mode. This enables an extra menu option of Import Searches on the Search menu.

2 Select Searches – Import Searches.
3 Find the correct drive, directory and file name – audit files have the extension .aud – and click on OK.

Importing the Clinical Audit search.

National Service Framework

Coronary Heart Disease
    CHD Existing – Investigations
    CHD Existing – Monitoring
    CHD Existing – Therapy
    Evidence of Arterial Disease – Investigations
    Evidence of Arterial Disease – Monitoring
    Evidence of Arterial Disease – Therapy
    High Risk Factors – History and Therapy
    High Risk Factors – Monitoring

The clinical categories for the new Clinical Audit CHD searches.

Make CHD reminders active

Reminders can automatically be generated for patients found as part of the monthly statistics. Reminders are simple text messages, aimed at practice staff, particularly clinicians, which will pop up within Consultation Manager when a patient in the audit group is selected.

The NSF CHD audits have some reminders built in to them, currently inactivated (pale yellow). These can be activated by the practice when you see the result of your audit.

Simply right mouse click on the icon ⬚, for example by 'Patients with Existing CHD with No smoking status recorded last year', select Reminder and click Active.

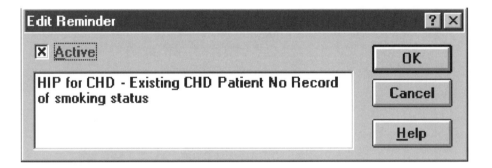

Generation of the NSF audits

Once you have loaded an audit onto your system, you can then generate the statistics for the previous month.

1   Access the Clinical Audit module. The Generate tab will be coloured red.
2   Click onto the Generate tab. Check the box Generate Reminders in order to generate reminders.
3   Start generating by clicking on the button at the bottom of the Generate tab – Generate data for [month/year]. If this is hidden, you may have to drag the lower horizontal lines up the page – point to the lowest divider line, click the left mouse and drag the divider line upwards.

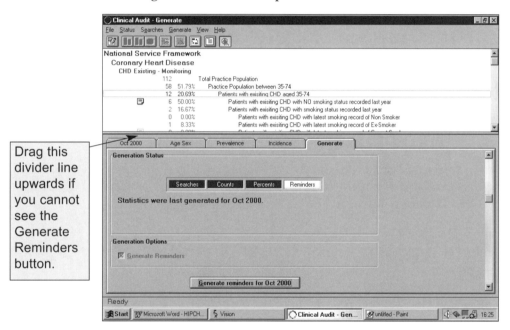

4   Once the generation has finished, the red Generate tab title turns to black. Underneath the four small windows of Searches, Counts, Percents, and Reminders, is displayed the most recent generation, for example, 'Statistics were last generated for Oct 2000'.
5   The new statistics will be available against each line in the upper frame.
6   When you select any patients found in the audit groups where reminders are attached, the yellow post-it reminders will be displayed when you select the patient.

Problem orientated approach to chronic disease registers

Why create a problem?

This section will help you to create a Problem Orientated Medical Record (POMR) for all those patients with evidence or risk of CHD according to the HIP NSF for CHD.

This will pull together *all* the diagnostic and other clinically relevant data for the patients who are at risk within your practice, and aid the collection of relevant and accurate data for audit purposes.

To create a problem for patients with evidence or risk of CHD

Once the NSF CHD Clinical Audits have been generated, a large number of groups will have been created. These can be found in the Patient Groups module.

All groups generated by the Clinical Audit module commence with a $ followed by AUD ****** or SUB ****** where the * represent a unique number generated at the time of the audit generation. The $SUB files are the Sub-groups of the audit and the $AUD files are the Main Groups.

Note Populating the problems should be completed each month in order to keep your POMR and CHD register up to date.

1 Go into Patient Groups module and locate the $AUD****** group 'All Patients with evidence or risk of CHD for NSF'.
2 Highlight the group and make it into the work group by clicking on ⊡ or select Group – Make Work Group.

3 Save the work group by clicking on the disk icon 🖫 and give the new group a name and appropriate description.
4 Exit the Patient Groups module.

Patient groups: making the Clinical Audit CHD group into the work group.

2 Highlight the group and make it into a work group by clicking on the 'blue blob' ⬤.

3 Save the work group by clicking on the disk icon 🖫 and give the group a name and appropriate description.

5   From the VISION front screen, access Modules – Populate Problems.

```
┌─────────────────────────────────────────────────────────────────┐
│ Populate Problems                                        ? X      │
├─────────────────────────────────────────────────────────────────┤
│ ┌─Source Group────────────────────────────────────────────────┐ │
│ │                                                   ┌─────────┐ │ │
│ │   Name:        NSFCHD                              │ Select  │ │ │
│ │                                                   └─────────┘ │ │
│ │   Description:  Pts With Evidence Or Risk Of Chd For Nsf      │ │
│ │                                                   ┌─────────┐ │ │
│ │                                                   │  View   │ │ │
│ │                                                   └─────────┘ │ │
│ └─────────────────────────────────────────────────────────────┘ │
│ ┌─Problem to Create───────────────────────────────────────────┐ │
│ │                                                   ┌─────────┐ │ │
│ │   ☐ Currently Relevant                            │ Define  │ │ │
│ │                                                   └─────────┘ │ │
│ │   ☒ Make Problem Currently Relevant                          │ │
│ │                                                               │ │
│ │   Event Date:    13/11/2000                                   │ │
│ │   Clinician:                                                  │ │
│ │   Read Code:     Coronary heart disease risk                 │ │
│ │   Short Name:    NSFCHD                                       │ │
│ │   Description:   Evidence or risk of CHD for NSF             │ │
│ │   End Date:                                                   │ │
│ └─────────────────────────────────────────────────────────────┘ │
│ ┌─Options──────────────────────────────────────────────────────┐│
│ │                                                                ││
│ │  ◉ Overwrite Existing Problem if Present or create if not Present││
│ │  ○ Add To Existing Problem or create if not Present           ││
│ └────────────────────────────────────────────────────────────────┘│
│              ┌──────────┐    ┌──────────┐    ┌──────────┐        │
│              │  Create  │    │  Close   │    │  Help    │        │
│              └──────────┘    └──────────┘    └──────────┘        │
└─────────────────────────────────────────────────────────────────┘
```

6   In the Source Group section, chose the group you created from the Patient Groups module.

7   Under Problem to create, remove the tick from Currently Relevant and click the Define button.

8   Fill in the Problem screen as shown opposite, making sure the short name is exactly as shown – NSFCHD.
     The Read Code '388A Coronary heart disease risk' was a new addition to the Read Dictionary in the Quarter 3/2000 update.

9 Under the Options section, choose 'Add to existing problem or create if not present'.
10 Click Create. The program will run through each patient with existing CHD and add a problem to their record.

Guidelines

Import the CHD Guideline and Report

The NSFCHD Guideline and Report are on the CD. Download them first. Then, within Consultation Manager, click on Select Guideline, then click on Import. Select nsfchd.txt and click on OK.

This will open the NSFCHD Guideline.

Now import the Report – from the Select Guideline screen, click on Import and select nsfchdr.txt.

The index mnemonic is NSFCHD. It can be accessed more easily if you add it to your Local Guideline Index by editing U_INDEX: Local Guideline Index: View the U_INDEX guideline, click on Design Maintenance icon [icon], click on the last line, then click on the Embed icon [icon] and type NSFCHD. Click on Save [icon] and exit. Repeat for the NSFCHD Report.

What the CHD Guideline contains

The NSFCHD Guideline should help your data entry for these patients. Within the Guideline are areas for display of current data and data entry templates. This will encourage data to be added within the Read Code hierachies defined by the Health Informatics Program and therefore improve the audit capabilities.

A separate NSFCHD Report allows a patient's data to be easily printed.

The NSFCHD Guideline.

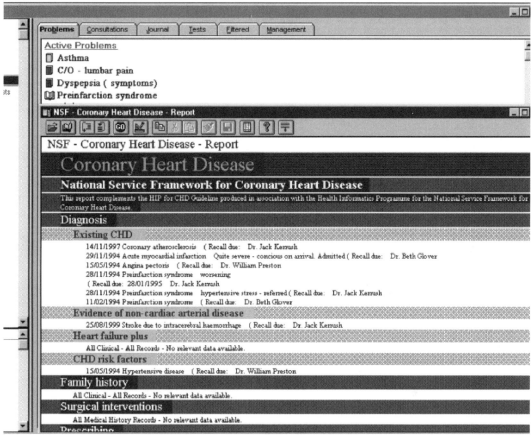

The NSFCHD Report.

Add Read Code triggers

What we suggest you do is set up triggers for this Guideline. Although this is optional, we strongly recommend it and overleaf we explain what happens when you do.

1 From the Select Guideline screen, type NSF and press Enter.
2 Highlight NSFCHD, and click on Triggers.
3 Click on Practice Settings first. It is important to change this from User settings *before* you enter the Read Code triggers as you cannot swap afterwards.
4 Leave 'Include children' checked.
5 In the top left window, type the first Read Code preceded by #, for example, #388A, then press Enter, then press Add. Continue down the list as illustrated. Make sure you include '388A Coronary heart disease risk'.
6 Finally click OK.

What happens once the Guidelines have triggers

This depends on how you have set up your Consultation Manager Options – Management.

For patients with a problem with any of these Read Codes, if your options are set to passive or active triggering of Guidelines, then when you select the patient, the NSFCHD Guideline is triggered – minimised at the bottom of the MRO column if set to passive. Click on the minimised Guideline to display it in full under the Management tab.

If you make an entry of any of these triggering Read terms so that the Guideline is triggered, *and* the patient already has a problem with the mnemonic of NSFCHD, then you will be prompted to open the problem (if semi-automatic problem generation is set) or the problem will be opened (if automatic is set).

If you are using problems manually, then before adding data to the Guideline first go to the Problem tab and open the problem 'Evidence or risk of CHD for NSF'. This ensures that any data added to the Guideline will also be placed under that problem heading.

Appendix B
The web site

The web site

The web site is available at:
www.radcliffe-oxford.com/edr
   At its launch, the site will include links to:

* PRIMIS
* NHSIA
* NICE
* NSFs for CHD
* Information on GPIMM and TNAMM
* The Virtual Library
* The Department of Health
* Software Suppliers and their user group web sites.

And it will aim to be a dynamic resource as this is a topic which is certain to change rapidly!

Appendix C
Health Improvement Programme for Coronary Heart Disease protocol in EMIS (Summer 2001)

EMIS has developed a module integrating with the clinical system that aims to assist in the data collection for the Health Informatics Programme for CHD. The programme is funded by the DoH and assists in the building of electronic disease registers, or 'virtual' registers as the programme calls them.

Once loaded by EMIS a separate section is available in the protocol menu for National Service Framework protocols. Familiarity with the protocol can first be gained by using it against a test patient, before activating for use by all the clinical team.

Support information and explanations of the programme structure and usage are included in the protocol menus. To see the protocol from the EMIS main menu:

DT = dictionaries and templates
C = codes, templates, protocols
C = NSF and clinical protocols.

There is then an additional menu:

N = National Service Framework protocols (EMIS/HIP)
S = standard practice protocols (access to the usual EMIS protocols).

On selecting option N, the further menu offers choices to activate, deactivate, try against a test patient, place in the access screen and to see and determine Read Code 'triggers' that will cause the protocol to run. This means that a number of codes can be set to start the protocol – a useful feature. Codes on the trigger list can be added or deleted to suit the practice.

On running the protocol there are 14 initial choices, related to clinical care, additional information on the NSF CHD guidelines, related patient information leaflets, etc. The data set used in the HIP for CHD is included under the section 'HIP for CHD information' and offers additional details of the programme design and implementation.

The data set is divided into 'Essential', 'Desirable' and 'Optional' and can be used as outlined in the book to assist in the coding strategy for the PCG/T.

Incorporating the HIP for CHD as a protocol is an advanced use of the EMIS system and will help with the clinical governance agenda.

Index

accidental damage 40, 41, 42, 47–9
accountability
   to PCG/health authority 59
   systems 57
analogue data, cf. binary data 11–13
Ash Tree House Surgery, policy
      implementation 73–91
audit
   clinical audit 6, 59, 135–9
   EMIS 96–8, 101–8
   Fylde PCG case study 96–7
   NSF CHD clinical audit 135–9
   policies, establishing agreed 64, 66
   policy implementation 68–70
   repeat 96–9
audit questionnaire, GRIM 48–50
automation phase, technology 10

behavioural variation, clinical information
      58–9
benchmarking, policies, establishing agreed
      64
binary data, cf. analogue data 11–13

capability maturity model (CMM) 22
case studies
   Fylde PCG 53–9
   risk management 44–6
case study practice 28
change, managing 21–50
CHD improvement
   audit, EMIS practice 101–8
   future, CHD coding 111–24
   Fylde PCG case study 53–9
   policy implementation, EMIS 93–108
   policy implementation, VISION 67–71
CHD register 114–16
chronic disease registers, problem
      orientated approach 140–3
clinical audit 6, 59
   NSF CHD 135–9
   see also audit
clinical coding, and clinical governance
      112–13
clinical governance 5, 56
   and clinical coding 112–13
clinical information, organising 57–9
CMM see capability maturity model
coding
   agreeing 119–24
   clinical coding systems 13–14
   crucial issue 11–13

GPIMM framework 25
inconsistencies 99
NSF CHD 119–24
policies, establishing agreed 61–6
reasons for 13
see also Read coding
communication
effective 58–9
information 68
computerisation
GPIMM framework 25
risk managing 39–44
computerised practice, risk management
44–5
computerised systems, cf. paper-based
systems 3–4
computers, problems 7–9
conclusions 125–7
cost benefit, IT 10
CTV3 version, Read coding 16

data analysis, VISION 90–1
data collection 56
EMIS practice 96
data entry, VISION 81–4
data integrity problems 50
Data Protection Act 94
database management systems 4–6
deliberate damage 40–2, 47
development stages, technology 9–10
direct replacement phase, technology 9

electronic disease register (EDR), schematic
6
Electronic Patient Records (EPR), GPIMM
framework 25
EMIS practice
audit management 104–8
auditing 96–8
CHD audit 101–8
Fylde PCG case study 99–101
integrating policy/computer system 95–6
policy implementation 93–108
Read coding 94, 96–8, 103
target population 101–8
EPR *see* Electronic Patient Records

errors, risks due to 40, 41, 43, 47–9
evaluation, policies 65
evidence-based guidelines/protocols 6
extended use phase, technology 9

filtering data 4–5
Framingham risk score
EMIS system 117–18
primary prevention 116–18
further resources 129–46
future, CHD coding 111–24
Fylde PCG case study 53–9
audit criteria 96–7
EMIS system 99–101

General Practice Information Maturity
Model (GPIMM) 21–36
and CMM 22–4
levels 24–5
practice profile 28
questionnaire 25–9
and risk 39–41
General practice Risk Information
Management (GRIM) 46–50
audit questionnaire 48–50
GP perspective 54–6
GPIMM *see* General Practice Information
Maturity Model
GRIM *see* General practice Risk
Information Management
guidelines
CHD Guideline and Report 143–6
VISION 87–90

hacking 42–3
health improvement programme, CHD
protocol 149–50
Health Informatics Programme (HIP)
135–9, 149–50
Holland House Surgery, policy
implementation, EMIS 93–108

ICD9/10 coding 13
identifying, 'at risk' patients 5, 17
ignorance, risks due to 40, 41, 43, 47, 49
IHD (ischaemic heart disease) 16–19

implementation, policies *see* policy implementation

improvement plan, policy implementation 70–2

improvement, policies 64

In Practice VISION Practice, policy implementation 73–91

inconsistencies, coding 99

information
  clinical 57–9
  communication 68
  NHSIA 112
  in primary care 7–8
  sharing 8, 68

information management, myths 8

information technology (IT), cost benefit 10

inherent risks 40, 41, 42–3

integration phase, technology 10

ischaemic heart disease (IHD)
  coding example 16–19
  computerised help 17–19

IT *see* information technology

Journal tab, VISION 79

learning phase, technology 9

limited use phase, technology 9

linked practice, risk management 45–6

Management Plans, VISION 85–6

Management tab, VISION 80

MIQUEST 55, 62, 112, 119

monitoring, policies, establishing agreed 65

multi-user systems, risk management 45–6

myths, information management 8

National Service Framework for Coronary Heart Disease (NSF CHD) 111–24
  clinical audit 135–9
  coding, agreeing 119–24
  data recording 118–19
  local policy, moving from 114
  VISION guidance 131–46

NHS Information Authority (NHSIA) 112

NHSNet 40

NSF CHD *see* National Service Framework for Coronary Heart Disease

opportunity risks 40, 41, 43–4, 48

organising clinical information 57–9

outcome, policies, establishing agreed 66

paper-based systems
  cf. computerised systems 3–4
  risk management 44
  steps to paperless systems 22–5

Patient Record View, VISION 77–84

Patient Reports, VISION 87–90

patients, identifying groups of 5, 17

PCG *see* Primary Care Group

performance improvement 59

personnel usage, GPIMM framework 25

policies, establishing agreed 61–6
  audit 64
  benchmarking 64
  evaluation 65
  implementation 65
  improvement 64
  monitoring 65
  outcome 66
  scene-setting 63

policy changes 7

policy implementation 67–71
  EMIS practice 93–108
  improvement plan 70–2
  In Practice VISION practice 73–91

policy integration, EMIS practice 95–6

POMR *see* Problem Orientated Medical Record

practice action screen, GPIMM 32

practice audit screen, GPIMM 32

practice case study, GPIMM 28–31

practice manager perspective, GPIMM 56–9

practice plan, GPIMM 31

practice profile, GPIMM 28–9, 33

practice profile over time, GPIMM 34

practice systems profile report, GPIMM 33

prescribing data, CHD register using 115–16

Primary Care Group (PCG)
  accountability 59
  CHD register 114–16
  future, CHD coding 111–24
  Fylde PCG case study 53–9

management information system 32–4
policies, establishing agreed 61–6
primary prevention, Framingham risk
    score 116–18
PRIMIS project 62, 112
problem orientated approach, chronic
    disease registers 140–3
Problem Orientated Medical Record
    (POMR) 140–3

questionnaires
    GPIMM 25–9
    GRIM 48–50

Read coding 11, 13, 14–16, 57
    benefits 55
    CTV3 version 16
    data entry, VISION 84
    EMIS practice 94, 96–8, 103
    history 15
    IHD example 16–19
    VISION 74–7, 87
    www link 15
recognition, identifying methods of 68
records, computerising patients' 7–19
resources, further 129–46
reward, identifying methods of 68
risk
    Framingham risk score 116–18
    and GPIMM 39–41
    GRIM 46–50
    identifying 'at risk' patients 5, 17
    inherent risk 40, 41, 42–3
    opportunity risk 40, 41, 43–4, 48
    risk assessment matrix 40–1
risk management
    case studies 44–6
    computerisation 39–44
    computerised practice 44–5
    multi-user systems 45–6
    paper-based systems 44

scene-setting, policies agreement 63
schematic, EDR 6
SEI see Software Engineering Institute

sharing clinical data 8
sharing information 68
SNOMED coding 13, 14
Software Engineering Institute (SEI), CMM
    22–4
staff competency profiles 35–6
    TNAMM 38
stages, technology development 9–10
steps, paper-based systems to paperless
    systems 22–5
structural variation, clinical information
    58–9
system usage, GPIMM framework 25
systems accountability 57

target population, EMIS audit 101–8
technology, development stages 9–10
templates, EMIS audit 107–8
TNAMM see Training Needs Analysis
    Maturity Model
training issues 7, 58
    policy implementation 68
    training needs matrix, GPIMM 35
Training Needs Analysis Maturity Model
    (TNAMM) 31, 34–8
    action plan screen 37
    audit screen 37
    competency profiles 38

viruses, computer 40, 42, 47, 49
VISION
    data analysis 90–1
    data entry 81–4
    guidance for NSF 131–46
    guidelines concept 87–90
    Journal tab 79
    Management Plans 85–6
    Management tab 80
    Patient Record View 77–84
    Patient Reports 87–90
    policy implementation 73–91
    Read coding 74–7, 87

websites 15, 112, 127, 146